The

Sacred

Language

Of The

Human Body

By Mona Delfino

TABLE OF CONTENTS

Dedicated to the memory

of Dr. John Jay Harper

and to the healing of humanity.

Acknowledgements

I would like to dedicate this book to everyone who ever touched my life, came across my path, and smiled at me in a public place without knowing who I was. I dedicate it to Spirit, the source of this book, and to everyone it reaches. You, the reader, are precious to me. If it wasn't for you, the world would be a little less curious, a little less caring, and a little less wise. Therefore, you are the star of the show. My gratitude goes out to all of those who supported me in writing my first book. I am grateful to all 5,000 friends on Facebook and Twitter, who read my posts daily and is still my friend!

My mentor who is gone from this world, Karen Land, deserves to be acknowledged for all of the 12 years I spent learning from this wise Cherokee healer.

My kids, Leah, Rachel, and Joshua, who have always been my best friends.

My sisters, Donna, Lucy and Cindy who knew I was a weird little kid and loved me anyway....

To all my loved ones who have crossed over into the other worlds, I love you and know you are here and there.

My dog Kita, who saved my life on December 15th, 2010, and to my deaf cat, Maya, who makes up for it by making me listen to her twice as much.

I want to thank Dr. Bernie Siegel, one of my dearest heroes throughout my life who spoke similar words of wisdom in the '80's when he was working so hard as a medical doctor and doing his best to tell the truth of life everywhere he went to all the people he touched, and still does. He touched my heart~

Dr. Norm Shealy, another fabulous doctor, the emeritus of medical intuition, who understood that we all need each other to heal. How blessed we are to have these incredible heroes in our world.

My editors, Sue Kay and Barbara Stott…thank you for asking me to take out all the little dots that became habit forming during the course of writing this book, and of course, for all your support!

I want to acknowledge my dear friend and client, Leslie Rushella, a beautiful lady who taught me how to write a book. Being from Jersey, thank goodness she holds absolutely nothin' back.

Doug Cristafir is one of the most talented Graphic Artists known to man, women, and every alien in the Universe! I have him to thank for the amazing book cover, my business cards, and my website. (Did I mention putting together this book as well?)

Last but not least, I dedicate this book to Pele, the Goddess of Hawaii. She taught me how to listen to the wind, watch, learn and live the magic of Aloha. She had her own courage to request a part in the book in 2009 because she loves people and wanted them to understand that love is what grows our world. Her fire purifies the heart of man, as she is truly a Goddess.

Thank you everybody; now let's get this party started! ~

ABOUT THE AUTHOR

I am Mona Delfino, a shaman by birth and overall, a very happy healer. As a medical intuitive, energy runner and healer for the last 30 years, I feel that putting this book out today is crucial with the amount of people I see shifting into who they truly are. In some ways, we might say this is a book of "Life 101" for people who are beginning to see themselves, and every person around them, going through immense change. In this book I will share with you a few experiences of when I was a kid so you can see that from the beginning, these teachings are from absolute truth from my heart to yours. All of the thousands of healings I have contributed to have made such differences in these people that I feel *now* is the time to share this knowledge and expertise with you to initiate understanding in our world that energy healing works. As far as I can see, this is what the future of health care is truly about, and may provide answers to many questions rising up around this dynamic topic. My feeling is strong about helping people discover their soul's true nature. I am skilled and certified in sound therapy, however I feel the intent of the human voice is the best sound therapist.

I have studied and had many opportunities to learn Indigenous ways, Native American and Hawaiian as well, along with several types of medicinal techniques.

My love for the Indigenous began when I went on a trip to Pago Pago, American Samoa in 1974. I was 16 years old when I sang and traveled with a musical group from Oceanside, California. We did a lot of performing, however the day we were asked to perform in our Sister City, Pago Pago, I felt like my world was complete! There were about 20 of us kids, and the second day we were invited to something very special. We were told that we would be going to see the home of an elderly lady and her granddaughter. Both had passed away many years prior, and little did we know when we arrived by bus to this house overlooking a very steep cliff, that this would be the adventure that started me on my way into healing and passion for the Indigenous for the rest of my life.

When we arrived and were still on the bus, we were told the story of the turtle and the shark. I remember being mesmerized by the beautiful tropical area on this gorgeous terrain as our tour guide spoke gently of the granddaughter and the elderly lady's eventual demise. She said that the two of them had told each other that if one was to die, the other would soon follow. The little girl wanted to be a turtle, and the grandmother told her she would be the shark. It was a type of contract that they set up, and one day it happened. The little girl was playing on the nearby cliff when she slipped and fell into the ocean about 200 feet down. The grandmother saw her fall and jumped soon afterwards to her death as well. The tour guide explained the importance of respect. She told us that anyone who yells loudly or becomes disruptive would stop the magic of what was to come. I was intrigued! She also told us that if we pointed our fingers or used a camera, we would be sadly disappointed. So off we went onto the land to the area of where the cliff met its end and where the ocean waves crashing on the rocks below had me hooked.

The guide began to sing in Samoan a beautiful song, (Malieh Telifah), and was throwing rose pedals into the water far below to lure the shark and the turtle to come see us. At this point my eyes must have been as big as saucers. Then it happened. The turtle showed up first in the waves as we gazed below. Within 5 minutes, the shark appeared with the fin showing, then making a little jump as it circled the turtle. It was breathtaking. I was in shock as I watched the most amazing thing I had ever witnessed. My heart felt as though it stopped beating…. Then one of the kids in our singing group pointed her finger and said, "There they are!" The turtle and the shark both went under the water and never came back up that we could see. The tour guide was absolutely correct. I was so amazed I didn't even have the urge to throw the girl over the cliff who pointed! From that day on, my life was changed. I would memorize that song and keep the memory always in my heart.

That was a myth or legend that was told in Samoa, and here we were so fortunate to see it as reality.

That same trip I developed a fever and almost died with a 106 degree temperature. Needless to say, our 1 week of singing became the trip of a lifetime for me and I would never be the same. My life began taking shape from there.

As I was finishing high school, I was also blessed to have been well received in another singing group called The Young Americans, which I was a part of for 2 years. When I turned 18, I received my first calling from Spirit. It was a feeling so undeniably strong that I had no choice but to follow it and see where it would lead me. That was when I moved to Northern California to live with my dad and eventually join the Jesuit Volunteer Corp. I worked 1 year as an activity coordinator for 4 senior citizen centers in Juneau, Alaska. I met my husband of 18 years 3 weeks before the end of that year when we married and had 3 beautiful children. My healing career began shortly after my babies were born.

~ IT BEGINS ~

As a child, many experiences lifted me into recognition of the path that was before me. I had what some people might call, a *sacred contract* with my brother Danny at 6 months old. My mother and siblings offered him the greatest of love, yet, Danny became worse physically in time due to a heart that was much larger than his little body could handle. He was the first heart transplant patient in Los Angeles at that age to ever have been operated on. Unfortunately, he did not make it. Fortunately, it brought me into awareness and I became alive with pure knowledge at 6 months old. I woke up to the spirit I am without age, without attachments, and physically and consciously became aware that I was back in a body. Looking and gazing at my hands, my inner voice was saying, "These will do." As I looked at the dresser, the curtains, the window, etc. I realized that I would need to remember this in order to eventually tell others, and mostly, my mother. The vivid memory of my grandmother coming into the room at that time and changing my diaper is as fresh within me now as it was 53 years ago. This is a direct memory with direct meaning from the time of this waking up process to where I am today.

At 6 years old I was sitting in my front yard playing with a blade of grass. I remember examining little hairs on this blade and remember asking myself how a tiny blade of grass could grow hair. Suddenly, my eyes went blind for approximately 2 minutes with bright white light. The neighborhood was missing from my vision. For a second, it crossed my mind that we might have been bombed as Los Angeles was having air raids in the early 60's, yet there was *peace* inside of me. I found out many years later that this was a *light experience* understood by mystics as an initiation into the world of mysticism. My memory from this moment forward would be sharp and aware as an observer. The schools

I attended, the animals we had, etc. would be in the forefront of my mind, yet I would only refer to these times if there was a reason to. I spoke to dogs and cats telepathically and I knew they could hear me. They actually spoke back, and the language they exuded was my language.

I used to walk to school with my sister and a friend every morning. I attended a Catholic school and wore a uniform. One day, my mom had changed detergents when washing this uniform that had me itching so badly that I lost consciousness during class in second grade. Instead of falling over, I transcended out of my body similar to a near death experience, however, I went into a trance-type state. I remember the teacher calling my name, and my continuous stare out the window was soon interrupted and back to my body I went. The tingling was too much as this reaction was profound. One thing it taught me was that I could transcend during any situation, yet stay remotely conscious enough to grasp what was happening at the time. This was the beginning of seeing my life as a mystic, or better yet, an observer. The best part was I learned I didn't have to attach to any outcome. Instead I could be larger in my spirit and still be aware.

Eventually, being present and focused became more magnified with the ability to transcend when necessary. I truly believe that within me, becoming the healer I am today was fed by this action. Mainly, I could see differently from others perspectives without attachment. As I got older I was quietly aware of true friendships. I watched certain people in my classes and discovered who was real and who wasn't. Somehow even at a young age, this seemed very important. I find childhood incredibly important for everyone because it's in these informative years that we make our minds up as to how we will be and what behaviors we take on when we get older. Now that we are in the time of changes in2012, I find most people have blockages in this area that are in the way of their spiritual growth. Mostly the age of 6 is where we determine our behavior through the decisions we make

—

8

for survival.

My passion, as I share this information with you, is to accomplish recognition from our childhood to where we are now. There has never been a better time to achieve everything we ever dreamed, to see our past and acknowledge it as just that, and realize that a new life means you discover yourself as a divine human ready to see life as an absolute adventure with Spirit, your ancestors, your guides, and the awareness that we are never alone. The acknowledgements I've carried are what excite me about sharing all of the truths I have found in humanity as each day brings in further growth for all of us to be a part of, to create with, and have each other to lean on. My clients have showed me huge parts of a global understanding; as they have taught me to not only see from a healer's insightful recognition, but also to listen beyond my own ears. This is what I feel has made me the healer I am today. What each person offers as they agreed to come in for their healings is making our learning more productive in this field of healing…not only in my office, but for the world.

I appreciate each one of you who are reading this book, and hope these insights of lessons learned and knowledge gained open doors for you. It gives me great pleasure to bring a different perspective with great understandings to the light of recognition for each of you, and more importantly, for our world to hear in this time of change.   Blessings, Mona~

1.

~ Conscious Health in a Changing World ~

"We are literally thought forms co-existing within the mind of God. If we apply this eternal Truth to our lives, we can peacefully co-exist with all life forms. This eternal truth stands here and hereafter…" *~John Jay Harper~*

We are in a changing world where awareness is beginning to lead humanity into more creative and responsible health. As individuals waking up to the dilemma in our health care systems, we recognize the need for change and realize that these times are highly significant for all of us. It's time to come together in unity and help each other to heal.

For thirty years, I have seen people search for answers to many of their questions regarding health in general. Fortunately, in my work as a Medical Intuitive Energy Runner, I have been able to tap in to the most important lessons a client is going through. This is cellular memory in action. When a repeated experience comes to the surface (We call it a "pattern"), then we are able to identify it and come to grips with it.

Our ultimate goal is to discover for ourselves a place inside where there is contentment, satisfaction, and peace. It is a place of surrender, yet empowerment. Most people are still searching, as day to day stresses are getting the best of us. Unfortunately, as this happens, our immune systems break down as our nervous systems get maxed. The adrenal glands become tired due to the constant thought processes and the "fight or flight" response kicks in. Sleep is interrupted and clear thinking can feel like a thing of the past. We tend to use up our energy on patterns associated with daily routines that are about how we think we are surviving or handling the demands of the day. For years, enlightened authors and positive speakers have spoken of meditation. Yet, if in our world, we do not seem to be able to find enough time to even sit down and eat, let alone meditate, how will we ever become healthy and stay that way?

~ LET TRUTH BE KNOWN ~

What we call "health care" today is actually an oxymoron. Simply put, I have yet to find health in this massive corporation where drugs rule, surgeries are at times unnecessary, diagnoses are out of line, doctors are busy with too many demands, costs are relentlessly criminal, insurance companies are denying claims, and last of all, our own lives have now been given over to someone who has no idea who you are.

On many levels, we know that this way of thinking about our health has been accepted and demanded for way too long. There are good doctors with very good hearts who generally would love to see a patient heal. However, even the best of doctors know that we are ultimately responsible for taking care of ourselves since they and their families also get sick and have to find answers. This is the way of life. Answers to illness are not found in prescription drugs. Most drugs stop your brain from associating what pain is and why it's there in the first place. Working with pain is doable with different forms of treatment; but when we drug ourselves, we obviously become dependent once again. In all the years I've worked in health care, I've seen that we have chosen to be submissive to others' ideas so as to not take responsibility for our own health. Heck, then we can even blame someone else if something should go wrong with the medicines we are taking. Take note of that word, "medicine."

~ UNREALISTIC MEDICATION ~

A Medicine Cabinet Life

One day I went to the spa downstairs from my office to soak in the hot tub after a long day of seeing clients. Suddenly I heard a woman's voice asking me if I was the Massage Therapist upstairs. I said, "Yes," wondering if she was going to ask for an appointment. Much to my surprise, she asked if she could talk to me privately in the sauna. She told me that she was on Prozac for six years. Her doctor kept her on it because it helped her depression. After about five years, she began to lose her memory. Soon after that, she was having trouble with her speech. Between her forgetfulness and then her slurred speech, she was sent to another doctor to be checked out with tests, etc. The doctors had diagnosed her with Alzheimer's disease and were ready to prescribe more drugs. Fortunately, her daughter was very aware that her mother was not one that she would have pegged for getting Alzheimer's. She insisted on her seeing an acupuncturist for her condition. The acupuncturist recommended that she go back to her original doctor and have her tapered off of Prozac, which her daughter then did. The agreeable doctor concurred, and within a few weeks, this woman was speaking normally. After a few months, she was steadily getting better. She wanted to tell me about it so that I could, in turn, tell my clients about the dangers of Prozac. This woman was in fine condition at the age of 62. This happened in the year 1992.

Statistics are something I take with a grain of salt. The same goes for medical studies. These studies change from one day to another, and there are thousands of people who are not included in statistics. No one can ever really know the truth of these tests; however, it isn't rocket science when we see the amount of prescription overuse in today's treatments. I read recently that prescription drugs, taken as directed, have killed over 200,000* people a year. I watched a program on television that stated that there are over 200 pill mills in Florida alone! These places dish out oxycodone, and people fly there to pick it up to sell it later. People are addicted, and people are dying. In truth, people are scared. People are ultimately lost and do not know where to turn. Some of the ones interviewed claimed they are needy for money and are in pain on many levels. We *do not* know all of the reasons for this crime being acceptable in our country alone; we *do* know that there are other cures, other options, and other places for people to seek help.

In this book, it is my passion to share what I have learned over many years working at a rate that most people would have a difficult time keeping up with, yet my passion for the work I have done and conditions I have seen, have led me to where I am today with the same passion I had when I began this work.

In 1998, I made an appointment with a doctor who was in charge of several clinics in the Mid-West. His family lived in my town and the wife and I were friends. I happened to be at their home one evening after telling his wife that I would love to talk to him. I had so much to share and didn't know what to do with all of this information that felt like it wanted to explode out of me. I found out that evening that he was a part of the National Institute of Health (NIH), making it even better for me since I was aware that Deepak Chopra was also a part of NIH. I went on to explain to this doctor that I had the ability, or "gift" as some call it, to know *why* a person comes down with an illness…no matter what it was. I told him that in order to get any form of illness or disease, you have to have a resonating factor somewhere inside you that makes you vulnerable to that condition in the first place. Hereditary information is a definite possibility, however if people understood that we are *not* our parents and have a different soul altogether, we wouldn't have to have any form of sickness, or even a heart attack, etc. if we were conscious of viewing life from our own eyes rather than someone else's. I figured since there was a part of National Institute of Health called "Alternative and Complimentary Medicine," this doctor might see the importance of what I was sharing and help me to find a way to teach them what I knew. These researchers could have a gold mine of information, respectively with understanding personality traits, etc. that cause illness in the first place. This information I had could help guide them into more knowledge for the sake of healing and quantum facts.

Unfortunately, the doctor looked at me strangely and proceeded to ask me why I had come to him. He wanted to know if I was looking for a grant. About that time, I began to feel as though no one would hear me. Bottled up inside me was a medicine cabinet of knowledge, and he wanted to know if a grant is what I wanted!

Saddened and disappointed, I made the decision to keep working as usual on clients and learn even more so that one day I could share it with the world. Well, today is that day. The timing was crucial and appropriate now, as more and more writers and speakers are addressing the need to change this system we call "health care."

In the last year, I have been acknowledged by many people, as my information has been getting out with the articles on my website, etc. I recently have been on five radio shows with great responses. More importantly, with one radio program, I was asked by the host how I saw the future of health care. My answer was, "By healing each other, of course!"

The radio host denied that this could work, and actually thought it would be humorous to make fun of me. He indicated that our country would never go for this and would never allow the *powers to be* to stand down for any reason. He commented that the world would never accept that simple concept. Again, my response was, "Never say never." If more people understood that we are all energy, pain is energy, etc, they might understand that we make our own choices when it comes to our health. The only difficulty is that most people don't have a role model who understands the concepts of living that free us and lead us to real health. Health has to be considered as the whole unit. In the next few chapters, I will discuss these sacred concepts and truths for these changes to be understood and acknowledged. My Cherokee mentor of 12 years used to say, "All it takes is the desire to know and the desire to act in order to heal." I found this to be very true, yet also if we take the word *responsibility*, we will see that it's not a word that we have to fear. Many people fear what they see as responsibility because they feel as though they aren't good enough and might fail in a task, even their own healing. Responsibility alone will change our lives and the lives of others. The healing within us, once it is understood, will generate energy around you where others will sense you are healthy and they, too, will want some of that energy!

~ ENERGY TRANSFERENCE ~

I remember in 1993 when Deepak Chopra came out with one of the most profound books I have ever read. Ageless Body, Timeless Mind gave us a clear look at what this energy was all about. In the book he talks about different studies that were done in laboratories with rats. One study shows two cages each containing the same amount of rats. One cage of rats was given love. They were petted and talked to each day for weeks. The other cage of rats was left alone except to be fed. After about three weeks, both cages were given poison with their food. The rats that were left alone died. The rats that were given love and petted, etc., lived as though they were fed the same food as usual. With those rats, it was the transference of love that kept them alive.

We all know that alternative therapies are getting more popular by the day. It is now common for people to receive chiropractic work as well as acupuncture, massage, Reiki, and even flower essences (all of which are vibrational healing therapies). There are clinics for amino acid therapy, and many body, mind, spirit clinics for getting a whole body adjustment. All of these therapies have something in common. Unlike the medical profession, they all have an understanding of energy and even more importantly, energy transference.

When I was nursing, I was in a patient's room, and she asked me why I was a nurse in neurology. I told her I loved the work and enjoyed meeting people; it made my day go more quickly. I also mentioned that I had just finished massage school and received my license. She smiled and said, "I own a Diet Center. I would love it if you would come and work there doing massage. I could get you all the clients you needed." I have to admit that I was tempted by the offer. Telling my husband at the time was going to be a bigger challenge than taking the position!

Needless to say, I accepted her offer and started my massage practice in 1990. My very first massage client came in at 300 pounds. She was upset, yet she acted strong. Her frustration about her life, her weight and her brother taking charge in a family business had made her a bit jealous and angry. So I gave her a Mona massage and consoled her through the only wisdom I had to offer at that time. After the session was finished, she said a polite thank you, and we parted ways. That night I began to feel horrifically nauseous and dizzy. At first I thought I was getting sick. But how could something come on so fast when I was fine an hour before? As

I was trying to cook dinner for my family, I became clammy, and my emotions were heading through the roof. I wasn't myself at all. I felt angry, strong, and now I was really feeling sick. I curled up in a fetal position and went under the kitchen table and rocked. I felt crazy. My husband was thinking about calling someone for help. I told him to leave me alone. He did, and that night I cried myself to sleep. The next morning I was fine. No problems at all. My emotions were intact and I felt good. I realized I had put my family in a" tizzy" the night before, not knowing what was wrong with me. The rest of that week was good. Then I heard from the Diet Center that the woman who was my first client had made another appointment! Yikes! How could I tell them that I didn't want to see her? Rather than becoming a coward, I did it. I bit the bullet and decided to give it another shot. When she came for her session, she walked in, wearing a red dress. WOW! She was beautiful. Her hair was gorgeous, her make-up was pristine, and she had lost five pounds in a week! I almost gasped as I wanted to say, "What happened to you?" Instead I asked her how she felt and told her she looked stunning. She said she was happily grateful for the work we had done the week before. She told me that she didn't know what I did, but whatever it was, she was a new lady. Boy, did it show!

That was when I first realized that this is something that people wouldn't get in a hospital or even in a counselor's office. I actually felt honored. From then on, the transference became easier. I realized that as soon as I recognized that these strange feelings were foreign and not a part of *my* world, they had to be someone else's. This, then, became my new way of healing and helping others. I wasn't afraid of transference after that, even though it seemed I could have had a reason to be. I trusted that this was God's way of interconnecting all of us. We are all energy and we can pick up on people around us and even those in other places. It's like using a cell phone. We have connection when we are dialed in, but we can hang up anytime we choose. We wouldn't hang up on anyone during a conversation for the most part, so why would we ignore a client or a loved one in their moment of need? We are transducers. We are givers (transmitters) and receivers of light, love, information, and communication. When a student would come in and tell me that transference really bothered them and that they were too sensitive, I warned them about being in this profession and told them they might do better taking a nine-to-five job for now. However, they would still be sensitive and would still pick up on co-workers and family members, etc. It would be better to learn the lessons of self-recognition now for tools to have in your future.

I taught classes soon after and showed massage therapists how to overlap the transference effect and *still* feel normal after a long day's work. To be a very good healer, you feel the pain, the emotion, the hardness, the insecurity, etc. of the person you are treating. Buying it as ours only attaches us to that sensation, and that's what is overwhelming. If it isn't ours, we need to *feel* that so as to help the person we love or care for. We can still be individual and even stronger in the long run when we aren't afraid of listening with our own body. This alone is a healing. Actually, this type of transference happens all the time for us, whether we're aware of it or not. We better get used to this occurrence because the future will prove this to intensify.

We are being magnetized as the shift gets stronger in our solar system. It is also happening in our physical system. We are seeing more people getting illnesses that are unrecognized by our physicians. More conditions in the body are occurring to which doctors might say, "It's all in your head," especially if they can't find anything wrong. You can have low back pain and go in for an x-ray, only to find everything appears normal. At this point, due to our insensitive nature, does anyone even know that you hurt? Many conditions today will be due to a high voltage of frequencies that are lifting your old patterns and emotions out of the body. The cells are actually *crying out* for healing and for freedom! The increases of solar flares from the Sun are proving that our bodies are being affected as we let go of old patterns. These patterns have to come to the surface to express themselves after being hidden within us for so long. In other words, these flares seem to be raising our consciousness and awareness while confusing and overwhelming us at the same time. As the movie line says, "Something's gotta give." This is why the buildup of emotions seems to be creating havoc in sensitive people. However, we are actually becoming like metal filings or fragments being pulled into the light. In order to do this, we must be cleared out of 3rd Dimensional thinking and living. This clearing ultimately will be our best friend. The love of the Universe moves us into a new realm called Unity Consciousness; Unity eventually in our cells, in our lives, and in our world.

I am not religious by nature; I am Spiritual and encompass all races, creeds, religions, etc. However, a quote in the Bible has stayed with me for many years. When Jesus said, "Where two or more are gathered," I pondered this as a child. I knew many adults who were confused by it or brushed it off with their limited understandings and taught just that. Jesus, in my opinion, didn't mean anything lighthearted or airy-fairy. Every time he spoke, there was a tornado of information and meaning behind his words. So, "where two or more are gathered" became the most important message this teacher ever offered.

In healing, one person reads and recognizes what someone else is experiencing. Once this conversation, whether it is aloud or silent, is acknowledged, it becomes recognition of energy. Therefore, the releases from any form of communication happen automatically and can be healed, and new adventures are developed. This is what I call the "big bang." It is like an explosion of releases within us when we discover the a-*ha* moment…or a resonance of the truth within us. There are a million big bangs every day. So, when two or more are gathered, "two" can include anything, not just people. This is extremely important for the future of health care. We don't have to have a Master's degree in healing or in science. We just need the comprehension and the compassion for true healing to occur.

~ BEYOND LIMITATION ~

It has been reported in medical studies that the phenomenon of energy transference in hospitals, nursing homes, etc. has made an impact in our world. One story was of a woman named Claire Sylvia who was in need of a heart transplant. She was in the hospital, very weak and dying. The doctors had not yet found a heart for her and were still looking; time was very short. Much to their surprise, there was a phone call, stating, that an accident had just occurred, and a man on a motorcycle had been killed. He was a donor, so they immediately set her up for surgery and performed the transplant. Upon awakening, the nurses asked Claire if they could get her anything, and her response shocked everyone when she said, "Yes, I would like a beer and French fries." The man who had died just hours before this transplant had been at McDonald's getting French fries when he was hit on his motorcycle by a car. Not only was her response amazing but so was the fact that she never drank beer! Later she had written a book called <u>A Change Of Heart</u>. (That book was also forwarded by Bernie Siegel, M.D.)

This happened in my practice throughout the years as well. I had a client who had just lost her son to a motor vehicle accident. He was nineteen years old and loved to fly fish, drive his truck, and be with friends. He wanted to have a family some day with children. His mother loved him so very

20

much and decided to donate his organs when the time came for someone in need. Well, that time came. Her son's kidneys were given to a man who had been on dialysis for a while. When it came to his needing kidneys, he received them from the nineteen year olds donation.

A year later, my client received a letter from the man with her son's kidneys. He did not know this family or anything about what had happened, however, he did find out where to send this letter. Upon her visit to see me one wonderful day, she showed me the letter stating that the recipient of her son's kidneys felt like a twenty year old kid. He said he began fly fishing and felt surges of energy to be with his four children again. His gratitude was overwhelming, and he had to find where to send this letter. My client and I were both crying as she was reading it. I felt this beautiful connection was occurring right in front of us, and we were both so blessed to be able to share this with each other.

It was then that I *knew* that there were no boundaries whatsoever to energy healing. Quantum awareness would take place even faster now as my recognition to all healing was opened wider to all possibilities. I turned on the hose, if you will, and from that moment, I challenged any form of healing to become greater and more productive. I knew my healing work was strong. Now it was about to become stronger realizing that since this was so real and mind blowing, then what about other transplants and blood transfusions? I have seen it, felt it, and even healed it with clients. When we or someone we know receives a blood transfusion or any kind of transplant, it is clear that the recipient takes on the energies of the person donating. This is new to us, but since we have the recognition now, we can also understand that our intent for any transplant makes a difference when we see this donated organ or blood as a clean and purified living part in us or our loved one. We only need to put our focus and intent into the new part coming into the body. Instead of just having the surgery, transplant, or blood transfusion, we are more than capable of energetically changing any unpurified part to being purified along with trusting that all will go well. Just as Dr. Masaru Emoto wrote in his book <u>Water Crystal Healing</u>, we can heal ourselves through music, words, and a combination of images.

~ NATURAL WISDOM ~

The future of health care will have to be known as "living simply so others can simply live." Eventually we will not have a medical profession to run to every time we get a runny nose. We will not always have insurance companies to pay our bills for us, and we will not have accurate diagnoses to depend on for taking a prescribed medication.

We have become unconsciously lazy in our own care as a global community; however, times are changing quickly. People ARE waking up to seeing this. We are living more from the heart as we feel more with compassion. Our children are hearing and learning these concepts, and there are many parents who are listening as well. We are ultimately tired of the game. I see many people who are asking questions and taking back their power. They just need direction.

Honesty is the best policy. To truly heal from our patterns and our individual hurts and pains, by acknowledging where or how they got there, we can counteract the condition. We can even go back in time and train our minds to overcome the very things that hurt us in the first place. Hypnosis works for many people with this very same concept. We do not need to depend on hypnosis, either. Even hypnosis doesn't work for everyone because some have a sense of wanting to be in control and do it themselves. If that's the case, more power to them!

We are coming into Oneness as we DO have each other. Our ancients and Shamans who lived in tribes (and still do) represent natural healing. Not only do they know the power of this oneness, but also they respect it and live their entire lives by it. This is happening in the Oneness today. Soon we will begin to feel lighter as time continues to magnify us into higher realms on our planet. The future of health care is going to have to be simplified. Herbs we grow will be understood through the feeling nature of what they are saying to the body. We can interpret these energies just as much as when we read someone's energy field. Flowers will be for color therapy and as essences to take internally. We will have to learn to listen, to slow down, and to still our minds from the need for gratification. Remembering that health comes from knowledge and acceptance, we, as a community of people, will realize that we are all healers by nature. We are all empaths to some degree, meaning empathetic transducers. We have all been given the gifts of caring and of course, love. Once we understand this sacred language that our bodies provide, we too will be magnifying ourselves back into a world of grace, beauty, and ultimately, teamwork of healing together. This is how we can respectfully give back to the Universe what the Universe is giving to us. This, my dear friends, is how we live in and with Nature. It's a whole language of adapting to who and what we really are.

2.

~ Reconstructing Human Awareness ~

"Align each decision you make with the person you want to be. If you do, you'll always know what action will create what you want."~ Nick Bogatin ~

Many years ago, I saw an interview with the Legendary American Scholar, Joseph Campbell. Joseph was a man who understood the patterns in human behavior as he explained it to us through myths and storytelling. I was, needless to say, glued to the television at a young age as I watched him come alive with passion in the Bill Moyer's series called "The Power of Myth."

I wanted so badly to remember his words, his teaching, and his humor. I knew I could go back and buy the tape, but I chose to embody his wisdom. His teachings became the truth of my life, and I knew it. Back in the days of the late 70's and early 80's, few people (compared to today) understood these teachings.

He wrote a book called *The Hero with a Thousand Faces*. In there, he tells the story of *"The Hero's Journey."* It describes the typical adventure of the archetype known as the Hero…the person who goes out and achieves great deeds on behalf of the group or the tribe. Campbell explores the theory that important myths from around the world which have survived for thousands of years all share a fundamental structure called a "monomyth."

The mono-myth of the summary of his book is this:

"A hero ventures forth from the world of common day into a region of supernatural wonder. Fabulous forces are there encountered and a decisive victory is won. The hero comes back from this mysterious adventure with the power to bestow boons on his fellow man."

The number of stages and the summary of the steps are as follows:

"The Ordinary World":

Here, the hero is uneasy and basically unaware; however, this is the one introduced so that the audience can identify with his situation. The hero is being torn and a type of polarity is pulling him in different directions, causing a dilemma. This person does not know his potential or calling.

"The Call to Adventure":

From something rising up inside this person, his situation gets shaken. Pressure comes and the hero must face the beginnings of the change.

"Refusal of the Call":

This is known as "the reluctant hero." Fear of the unknown sets in and he tries to run from the adventure… however brief. In concordance to this emotion, a sense of duty, obligation, or even insecurity can bring in inadequacy. The hero wonders if there's danger ahead.

"Meeting with the Mentor":

Once the hero commits to the quest, he finds the teacher. A guide appears as a helper or even an ordinary man, who helps him on the journey to courage and wisdom.

"Crossing the Threshold":

The end of Act 1 demonstrates that this is the point where the hero crosses into the field of adventure and leaves the Ordinary World. He becomes better adapted to unfamiliar values.

"Tests, Allies, and Enemies":

These are what the hero must undergo in order to begin this transformation. A new approach, the confrontation with death, and in a single moment, the greatest fear is faced, and out from death comes a new life.

"The Reward":

Treasures are won by facing death, however, danger still lurks as there could still be a belief that the treasure may become lost.

"The Road Back":

As the story is almost finished, the hero is driven to complete the adventure. He needs to revisit the mentor to learn new mentoring. Then he returns to the path he started on…reborn.

"The Resurrection":

The hero becomes tested again as he ventures on the threshold of home. By the hero's actions, after he encounters another brush with death, he becomes purified and reaches higher levels proving the lessons were learned.

"Return With Elixir":

The hero now returns home and achieves the goal of the quest. This elixir is not a plant or a medicine as we know it. It is the balance between the material and the spiritual world. Now there is freedom from fear and from fear of death. The hero is now transformed.

As you can see by the story itself, this may sound very familiar to you. For those of you that resonate to it, you can see that this is ALL of our paths that we are on today. We are, by right, our very own hero writing our very own book.

~ IT BEGINS WITH AWARENESS ~

When we think about "how" to begin to shift our thoughts, it must come first through a circumstance's occurring, and then being brought to our awareness for a reason. Awareness truly comes from the heart through emotions. Here are some ways to help you identify how awareness occurs:

1) A reaction we are having to a current situation
2) A frustration because we are not able to control an outcome
3) A very happy and enlightening moment with a friend, and then an awakening as to why we just became "happy"

4) A dream that encourages us to "feel" connected, whether we remember the whole thing or not
5) Hearing a song on the radio that triggers a memory of someone or a time in your life

I could go on about how awareness happens; however, the bottom line is that as we get our "A-HA" moment, it is important to acknowledge it! Since each of us has a different concept of what is important to our own growth, we can develop into our Self and allow these encouraging moments to take a priority in our consciousness.

In today's times, it's the little things that create a shift in perspective due to this awareness. We get so busy and caught up in our lives that we don't even take the time to

In today's times, it's the little things that create a shift in perspective due to this awareness. We get so busy and caught up in our lives that we don't even take the time to feel the moment happening. Meditation is meant to examine this on a higher level, but even that doesn't grasp the depth until you recognize it inside of yourself.

The concept of a moment seems so trivial when you think about it…But what's really involved in a moment that makes such a difference as to how we advance in our understanding of our Selves?
We can see how far we have come from our childhood. We can ask ourselves the question, "If I know I came out of elementary school a long time ago, would I want to go back to it when I was in high school?" Chances are, you'd say, "Of course not!" Well, if we answer like this, then we must admit that we see how far we've come….and how silly to even think that going back to elementary school was even an option!

The moment we lived back then, however, accounted for every detail that led us to high school in the first place. Moments are only the recognition of a perception that comes clearly, and then advances to the next one. So if this is the simple case, then what is stopping us from achieving more of these moments of recognition faster?

The answers to that are insecurities that are due to old fears. If we had no fears from prior experiences, (not just from this one life time) we wouldn't have any reason to "hold back" and our knowledge would be happening at such a great rate that we would have absolutely *nothing* stopping us from being everything we choose to be and become in our world today. Insecurities have been a part of life, obviously, for eons of time!! Fears are there on very subconscious levels for protection... but protection of what? Have we actually detached our Self to believe we were enhancing our Self, when really it's been fear all along?

So many people have believed they were doing the "right" thing in life for themselves through an action, and then they found later that somehow things didn't turn out the way they'd hoped. Why? They attracted an outcome through a level of fear without recognition. Many people would say "It was God's plan," or they were just not important and life took a course because they weren't good enough. It's amazing how we see ourselves and judge due to an outcome.

But that's our human limitation! If we have the ability to do anything, feel anything, and see in any way we want to, then what could possibly be stopping this amazing concept called "Sacred Sight"?

~ SACRED SIGHT ~

I looked in the dictionary recently to see how many definitions I could find under the word, *sacred*. There must have been over 30 definitions, not to mention the Bible quotes! One, for example, is the "Sacred Heart of Jesus." Sacred, in this case, is more of an adjective describing the purity of heart seen by many about Jesus. Just as this meaning arises, other definitions, such as "divinity," or even "holy" comes up.

I see this word as a reason to call something respectable. *A true respect* for the human body is how I revere it as sacred. So what would the idea of sacred sight mean?

When we look at a rock we realize that this rock has been here for eons of time. It became a rock simply through its own evolution. We might decide to use the phrase, "If this rock could talk." By using a phrase like this one, we could say that we SAW this rock as sacred. In other words, we are paying attention to the fact that we respect this rock and the years it has seen, instead of taking it for granted and not giving it any thought at all. This is what is known as Sacred Sight. When you are respectable to others, to any circumstance or situation, then in truth, you hold this awareness as sacred. You are the observer and are not interfering in their process. You see with your heart. This is how we begin to understand the concept of Sacred Sight.

Once we begin to allow ourselves to get to this awareness, we then can go deeper with the feelings of being connected to all things!! Native American tradition has taught this for thousands of years. Where did this ability within all of us get so caught up in separation? Being *one* with all things requires us to simply know that we are one with all things. It's simple because it's true. Many of us have seen ourselves separate from the Earth, the Ocean, Nature, etc. Some of us have done so out of, what we've considered, respect or awe, if you will. It's wonderful to know the "gratitude of the magnitude," however, power is *within* all. When we truly connect to our surroundings, we feel a sense of peace. I'm talking about feeling nature and its magnificence *within* ourselves. When we connect ourselves, then we become that same magnitude within, which holds the balance of expansiveness, completion, clarity, and divine purpose.

~ HEREDITARY GIFTS FROM EARTH ~

"Whatever does not exist in the body can't be found in the Universe. Whatever exists in the Universe can be found in the body." - Ghandi

In Gregg Braden's Youtube presentation on Consciousness, he describes how the magnetic fields of the Earth have been proven to be affected by events, such as 9-11…. only 15 minutes after the first plane hit the world Trade Center. Science has clearly documented these conditions of the human heart to reflect the spikes in these magnetic fields through satellite activity…. simply from our emotions! When we tune in to our heart's electromagnetic emotions, the Earth can hear us and aligns to this as well. If everyone had only anger and pain, the Earth would HAVE to act the same in order for us to see the mirror as a whole. It may be that we have to feel shaken to awaken. Or maybe we'll learn to advance from clarity this time. (Jesus would be so proud! :)

So if this is really the case of connection, we must be more cognizant of our responsibility within our Self *and* within the entire world! What a wonderful responsibility to have at a time most necessary in our world… what a feeling to know you and I are contributing to this magnificent purpose.

We've waited for years for others to come forward, and have cursed that which doesn't relate to our idea of love, or what we felt justified in. Why not become the example we want others to see, feel within ourselves, and get simplified? Again, it can be so simple.

There is a wonderful slide show that's been going around the internet since 1998. I just received it a few days ago, just in time to get it in the book!! It clearly is a wonderful piece of information about certain fruits and vegetables that resemble parts of our body. For example, when you slice a carrot, did you know that it looks like an eye with the iris and a pupil? Of course, carrots have Vitamin A that is good for the eyes!

The list continues….

Tomatoes: There are 4 chambers when you slice a tomato. The heart has 4 chambers. They are both red. Tomato's have lycopine. This feeds the heart and the blood.

Grapes: In the bunch, they resemble the shape of the heart. Alone they resemble a cell. Grapes are known as anti-bacteria cleansers in the body and are good for certain cancers.

Walnuts: These actually look like a brain! They have a wrinkled appearance, and it looks like they include cerebrums and cerebellums. Walnuts help develop more than 3 dozen neurons-transmitters for brain function. They even have a fold…creepy or not, it's true!

Kidney beans: Yes, they look like kidneys. They even help maintain kidney function.

Celery, Bok Choy, Rhubarb: They all resemble the bones. These veggies actually improve bone strength...Bones are 23% sodium, and these are 23% sodium. The skeletal system needs sodium to keep the marrow strong.

Avocados: These actually take 9 months to grow and ripen. Can you guess what they look like and what they're for? Avocado's balance female hormones and look like a woman's cervix. They've been known to help prevent cervical cancer.

Pears and Eggplants: These are similar to the avocado, but they look more like a womb. Their nutritional benefit is also important.

Figs: These hang by two's. Believe it or not, they've been known for helping increase sperm count in men, and help men to overcome sterility!

Sweet Potatoes: Ok, this one looks like a pancreas, and it helps to balance glycemic conditions related to diabetes.

Olives: Olives help with function and health of the ovaries... well, they kind of resemble them too.

Oranges , Grapefruits, and Citrus: These maintain the movement of lymph to and from the breasts. They also represent the mammary glands!

Onions: These are like the body's cells. Eating onions actually helps the body in the way that an anti-biotic does. They clean waste from a cell. Onions also produce tears, which washed the tissue around the eye. Its cousin, garlic, has very similar effects on the body's immune system.

Of course, these are only to name a few. How fascinating it is when we pay attention. I don't know about you, but it makes me love our Earth Mother more all the time.

Herbs, no matter what part of the world you are from, have been known to heal the body for thousands of years. There are 4,000 herbs in America being used to cure conditions in our systems… and that's only the "known" ones. I have never picked up or held a plant without it telling me what it does. It relates through the same means as the body. It gives your body its language for you, just by holding it in your left hand and by you feeling the sensation. Since this is our receiver side, there is nothing we can't determine as "good for us" just by holding it directly and getting the result in your body. If we can connect this strongly with osmosis of other life forms, just think of all the things we could be missing out on? What about the animal kingdom? We have heard of having a totem animal. How is it we can relate so well to a cougar, an elk, a rabbit, etc. and then not get the sense that all things are connected? Again, another reason to acknowledge how we can change our world by working together and considering health care from the heart… we sure have waited for it… I'd say for over 2,000 years.

Our part in this world is exceptionally and integrally important, and what we do with it makes a difference. How you live it day by day, and what you do with it, is totally up to you. The "drop in the water" effect is happening second by second. Our words, our thoughts, our perceptions, and our actions are all changing this world… seconds at a time.

~ TRANSFERENCE HAPPENS... ~

As I know how important it is to read the body, I can tell you that healers with this capability are profound in the here and now, and for our future in the profession of healing!

I remember when I first received my massage license!! The excitement was almost overwhelming because I had worked to pass that test to the absolute best of my ability, and man...what a test!! If you haven't taken a massage therapy course, you would never have an idea of how difficult it really is! You really need to know your muscles, insertions, counter muscle, etc...

I had quit my nursing job to do this full time, and you can imagine knowing you were ready now to follow your passion. Oh boy!!!

I started out renting a small space behind a diet center. The excitement was almost overwhelming because I knew this was it! I even quit my nursing job, without telling my husband at first, because I was SO ready to help others the way I saw healing could be... absolutely personal!!

Then my first client scheduled through the diet center. I was all gussied up and ready to do my job... when I was taken by a huge surprise... she was suicidal.

Her anger of being overweight and "not good enough" had really made that Goddess part of her turn to despair. She shared with me the upsets and frustrations as I was working on her body. Little did I know that as we were in this space, I was taking on her pain. It wasn't so much physical, it was mostly all emotional. Needless to say when I was done with the session, I began to feel sick to my stomach. Fortunately, I had no other clients and decided to go home. That night, I threw up several times. I also had the feeling that I wasn't "me" anymore...more like I wanted to sit under a table and just rock myself back and forth. It was very disturbing not to be able to gather yourself… most importantly, I remember feeling that maybe I would be insane and not come out of it…and what would happen to my kids??

I had help going to bed by my husband at the time. (who fortunately didn't call the men in the white coats) I woke up in the morning feeling just fine. No hangover from the energy of that woman… maybe I'd be ok?? Whew! What a relief!!

Then I went to my job again to find out she had called to make another appointment 2 days later. YIKES! Do I cancel? Do I tell her she needs to see someone else? Do I consider crushing her by telling her I don't want to see her? Well, after the initial scream from the inside, I calmed down and told myself that if I got through this one, I could do it again… maybe.

The day came, she showed up, and WOW! She had changed her hair to a different style; she bought a new dress and was wearing it, and even lost a couple pounds! What just happened?

When I massaged her, she felt better, more peaceful, and she even laughed at one of my silly jokes! She then gave me a huge hug and said she'd never felt better! Good! I really didn't want to tell her I felt like absolute…you know what …that night!

The truth is, that lesson was for me. Once I was able to get through the initial chaos of transference, I could go about realizing that maybe this was normal, and everyone who did healing work feels this?

Anyone who does any healing work, no matter where you come from, race, religion, etc., feels the person they care about…one way or another. This is truly natural for everyone, but maybe not at the level I ran into from the start! (Thank God or we'd be in a world of hurt!) Transference is strictly the combined energy of the knowledge that we all are *one*. It's osmosis in action.

~ HOW DO WE KNOW? ~

So often, students have asked me how they would know if how they felt after being around someone, (talking to them or working on them) belonged to them or the other person.

There are different answers to this question.
1) Did you feel this way before you had the encounter?
2) Is the way you're feeling related to a mood that you go through on a regular basis?
3) Does it feel foreign?
4) Do you hurt in a place you didn't hurt before you had this encounter?

These are some of the ways you can identify if this is transference. Simply put, recognize it could be someone else's pain, emotion, or even their thoughts and take the guilt off you.

Transference happens in our own homes. When our kids are sick, we take on their illness so they don't have to suffer. Most parents don't even know this happens! Or the child will take yours so you don't have to experience it. (Here we thought it was just contagious!) Have you ever been around anyone with head lice for just a moment and then started itching? That's an obvious example; however, take that to larger levels, and you'll find there's much more we don't realize. The thoughts of your friends or partner can influence your very own thought process, and turn you into who they are, rather than who you are in any given situation. This is no different then when we see our high school kids perform under peer pressure. We, as adults, usually don't see it for ourselves.

Another interesting point when it comes to health is related to parents. When we were growing up in our parents' home, we didn't know that, for the most part, we wanted to be pleasing and accepted. Most of us didn't understand why we didn't meet the grade with our moms or our dads. (This is why counselors ask you, "Did you get along with your mom?) Typically, we eventually take on the behavior of our parents in one way or another without realizing it. This, too, is natural. Dr. Bruce Lipton, author of _Biology Beyond Belief_ and most recently, _Spontaneous Evolution_, talks about the environment being our difficulty relating to clarity within ourselves. That includes the sub-conscious belief systems we carry within us that do not actually belong to us; maybe they were our fathers belief that we had to work hard to make a living. Therefore, if we lose our job, we feel as though we have failed and cannot see that we possibly will be given a new position to use our talents differently. This is what our home environment was like. We chose, on some level, to buy into the concepts of our families and our peers… not taking full responsibility for our own truth.

In our world today, it's important to ask yourself if the feelings you feel and the way you react is yours… or theirs?

The reason I bring this up is because when it comes to our health, we ALWAYS have choices in our responses, our actions, our reactions, etc. (Life would be so boring, actually, if we were clones!)

Doctors tell us that when we enter their office, we must fill out a form about ourselves. The first question is usually, "Are your mother and father still alive?" Then, "Does anybody in your family have heart problems?" This list goes on so the doctor can get to know your bloodline history.

~ BLOODLINE "HAND-ME- DOWNS? ~

When we talk about patterns in the body, we need to understand that these are changeable. If they weren't, we might as well curl up and tell ourselves that we are doomed and life isn't worth living!! Ugh.

In the medical profession, we have understood that disease can come from hereditary bloodlines. When they talk about heart disease, MS, diabetes, or even cancer, you are automatically at risk. From the Medical Intuitive perspective, this is true to a point. The reason it's true to a point is because we take on our parents' behaviors and actions, and this can cause the same effect in your blood as they have/ had. But this isn't the case for everyone obviously. So we live in fear of the unknown, wondering if we will end up just like them. We get a jittery feeling from nerves and immediately wonder if a heart attack is coming on.

All we need to do is realize that if the behavior(s) of our parents are a part of ours and we haven't dealt with them, then we need to take a good look at them and decide how we are going to shift.

You know how we laugh when we hear someone say, "OH no!! I'm becoming my mother!" Usually it's because we get that lovely A-HA moment when we hear ourselves talking just like she would or acting a particular way toward …housecleaning. The real truth of the matter is that we learned what we didn't like about our parents and vowed to never treat our children the way they treated us, right? So if this is the case, then when it comes to our attention, we will recognize it and shift it immediately as to not allow that part we didn't like to interfere in OUR life today. This is important in how we see the word *hereditary* in our lives. Sometimes the behavior is harder on us than the disease! Also, be careful about judging yourself too closely. This can also have the effect of bringing it on because at that point, it becomes fear-based.

So hereditary bloodline comes from the energy of the reason a disease is there in the first place. Cause and effect are in action. This can always be changed, rectified, or even shifted in minutes once the A-HA moment becomes effective.

It's absolutely amazing today to know this type of understanding in transference. We need to remember that genes are just as mutable as water. There is nothing anywhere that claims that every single person will some day be doomed in life because of their hereditary background. If all things are energy, then we could honestly say that we are in charge of this. My mentor of 12 years, who was a Cherokee Healer and seer of the body, used to say that there is no such thing as a miracle… it's just lack of knowledge. If you stop and think about that in today's world of Quantum Physics and Science, I believe we would find that true.

3.

~ Diagnosis vs. Condition ~

"The simple truth is that generally happy people don't get sick." - Dr. Bernie Siegel M.D.

America is still a country that seems to be misdirected when it comes to health care. This is disconcerting when we can't even afford co-pay, let alone, a doctor bill. Heck, some of us are even having trouble with paying our mortgage!

In the past when it was thought that doctors knew best, it certainly didn't seem intentional that doctors diagnosed cases that may not be what the patient had at all. As a matter of fact, it's happening today that more and more physicians are finding that patients have more emotional problems that relate to the physical ailment. However, the solution is still at bay for the physician, unless they can solve it with a pill or surgery.

In my 25 years of reading clients' energy fields, seeing eight people a day for 15 years alone, I have found nearly 500 misdiagnosed cases. They ranged anywhere from a muscle sprain to a serious heart condition. Some of the cases were diagnosed through a side effect from another drug. I do not like the term *diagnosis* mainly because this word represents that you are now labeled. If people think that it's better to have a diagnosis, that's fine, however, it might feel better if we were able to see what might be ailing us through knowing rather than guessing. Bernie Siegel M.D. has often stated that doctors do not really know what the matter is with you, and to live life well, you are best to remember who the true healer is. Of course, it's you. There are so many alternative therapies today that can offer help and suggestions for healing, and these therapies do not have to cost an arm and a leg. With so many people without health care insurance or even jobs for that matter, the time has come to allow for more understanding through simpler and less expensive means.

Diagnoses are sometimes very difficult to call. One diagnosis can have several different symptoms. As a matter of fact, there are so many symptoms that mimic each other that it's hard to diagnose just one label sometimes. For example, a stroke has similar symptoms as a heart attack. In today's world, there are too many unique cases that even doctors are confused as to what label they should hand to a patient. Personally, many clients concur that these are conditions occurring in the body, and that's what needs to be seen as the effect, not the cause. I worked with a neurologist for a few years who said over and over that people with headaches and migraines were the hardest to work with. He said there were many different reasons why a patient gets headaches, and as a physician, even he didn't know the best remedy to prescribe. When I suggested to him that the patient is confused about making a decision, and possibly needs to hear that, he laughed. However, I didn't find it a laughing matter. That is why when I did hands on work with my clients, they learned that, not only were they in a state of having to make a decision, but if a migraine would be persistent, I informed them that this is when you know what decision to make, but you just aren't making it. It certainly isn't a fault; it's just knowledge that I read and deliver. Nine times out of 10, the client not only hears it, but then allows the healing to take place because the cause resonates to the truth, and then the headache doesn't seem to come back. THAT is energy working through bio-feedback of truth.

We are going through a period of time right now in our world where to be able to *start* to heal, we can apply simple measures. Going back to our values, such as being a good listener, remembering that we were once in the same boat as someone else, etc, gives us more room to understand and be compassionate toward our neighbor, loved one, or even co-worker.

A few years ago, a client on her death bed came in because the doctors she worked with couldn't find that she even HAD a problem! They just knew she obviously couldn't eat and keep down any food or drink. They ran several tests, of course, and nothing turned up on a scan of any kind. They were then baffled and told the woman's husband (after two months of her being in the hospital) that it must be stress. No diagnosis could be reached. She had had a car accident, landed in between the seat, and soon afterwards, found she couldn't eat without throwing up. Her husband came into my office frantic, carrying her in his arms and pleading for help. She had lost 55 pounds in two months…only being fed intravenously. We had not seen these people in our clinic before. The husband said he'd go anywhere that could help her because the hospital just discharged her and told him to take her home and make her comfortable… "There's nothing that can be done."

I don't take no for an answer very easily… so I had him lay her on the table. I took one look at her stomach from a distance and saw she had a small bulge at the base of her xyphoid process. To me it was obviously a hiatal situation… possibly a hernia. So, I massaged her stomach area, I listened as she cried, saying God was punishing her and that she must have done something wrong. I assured her God wasn't punishing her and that it could just be a small blockage that hadn't been located yet. Sure enough, the hiatal was like a rock and was cutting off her oxygen as well as her circulation and blocking the duodenum so that she couldn't eat. I simply massaged it in a downward position and had her take deep breaths. Her tears then slowed and a sense of calm came over her face. I told her she might try to eat watermelon and drink hot beef broth then come back in a few days. Three days later, when I arrived at work, a woman was standing at the door. I didn't recognize her. She was wearing make-up, her hair was beautiful, and this woman threw her arms around me, thanking me for saving her life.

"Oh wow!" I remember saying and asked her if she kept the watermelon down. Obviously, she did, and from then on, kept anything down she chose to eat! Within 2 weeks after that, she was gardening and enjoying riding motorbikes with her kids!

When we are diagnosed with *any* diagnosis, we have no idea what's really happening, except to believe what we've been told by someone who, according to American standards, should know what's wrong with us! After all, how else would we begin to recognize what was happening in our *own* body?!

It would be nice if we could self-diagnose, but we would need to really be in touch with ourselves to do this. Better yet, wouldn't it be even nicer if we didn't have to diagnose at all and actually feel symptoms occurring as a wake-up call and begin taking homeopathic remedies or herbs to help lessen the symptom while at the same time, take responsibility as we see fit? Maybe we could even consider that energy is a part of everything and therefore, understand some of the ways our body needs to let us know that we have to take a good look at ourselves. The physical body is our vehicle. It is also our mirror. We know this… so then, why do we *not* listen when it speaks to us? Something as simple as our eye watering could be that we haven't cried over something that is hurting us emotionally. Nine times out of 10 we didn't know something was there in the first place to cause that kind of physical reaction. When we have a stomach ache, for example, is it just that we must have caught a bug? Is it possible that we have been going through heavy changes and not dealing with a situation that calls it to our attention? When the body is sneezing, we automatically think that we have an allergy. Allergies are usually because of poor digestion in the first place. Maybe the body is just clearing out from a toxin that it came in contact with. Also, when we have a condition like a cold, this is not because we caught one. It's because we either needed a break and we knew it or we are facing a confusing dilemma and feel overwhelmed. Not all symptoms have to be devastating if we consider everything has a reason. Because we are sensitive beings and our body is our vehicle, would it make sense then that this physical part of us would want to alert us to our deeper emotions? One thing I really learned working in the Medical field for six years was that everyone saw the body as a mystery and that it had to be something outside of us causing aches, pains, headaches, etc. God forbid, your first thought might be the "C" word! A blood pressure is an interesting metaphor to life. If we really understood that, we would be able to detect that the systolic number (the top) is about the stresses that are affecting you from the outside world. Your job, your routine, your kids always needing your attention, the frustration of being in traffic, etc. The diastolic number is related to the stresses on the *inside* that are not taken care of or recognized. This may include your concern for a loved one or afraid of getting a bad grade in college, not fitting in with friends or a number more reasons that cause a lesser- than reaction.

Is life really a crapshoot? We simply are not pawns to some matrix in the sky with no cause. In all things, there is always a *cause and effect*. An action brings a reaction. This is common sense of science. In the same way, nothing ever happens to any of us *without* a cause.

Some of these causes are based with fears, which, of course, lead to illness, scarcity, doubt, and all the things that stop us from our potential. What I've noticed most in people is their fear of not being good enough. This is huge... I would say it stands first in the world of "pain bodies." If someone has money issues and can never seem to get ahead in their eyes, they feel they did something wrong. If they get sick, they feel they did something to deserve it. If someone assumes that a person is whispering quietly to another, they automatically think they are talking about them. When a loved one dies, they feel "Did I say all the right things?" It's the shoulda, woulda, coulda syndrome. The list goes on and on around this issue. Truly, it becomes a self-created judgment and it puts us in an awkward position within ourselves. If you think of how our cells mimic our thoughts and behaviors, then what do you think will or might possibly occur in the body when these questions are asked and not dealt with?

~ THE CULPRIT....INSECURITY! ~

Through every person, there has been some form of insecurity that stands in our way of clarity. These are fears that become blockages on some level, preventing us from becoming free in ourselves. The opposite of this is confidence. Inner peace is what we are all seeking, and to get there, we must recognize what it is that continues these behaviors within us. Even though insecurity is an expression of the lack of self-esteem, insecurity can be a TOOL when we recognize it, and it can lead us to the peace of confidence inside ...like a stepping stone. It brings up sensitivity, which then can transpire into compassion as we see ourselves learning through it. Being aware of our perceptions and recognizing them as such, we can change them in an instant.

We simply cannot escape the law of attraction however, or the law of cause and effect, so I've listed a few of these behaviors to help us identify these in ourselves:

Here are a few to ponder:

Denial, anger, lying, defensive behavior, manipulation, giddy, control, unrealistic ideas, the all-knowing behavior, quiet, submissive, dependent, co-dependent, escapism, overly emotional (drama queen or king), overly confident, constant fatigue, complaining, loud, irritating, overly talkative, ego, anxiety, opinionated, overly religious, etc.

I'm sure you can come up with a few of your own! It's fun to teach a class on Body Intuition and then have students come up with what they see as insecurities. These are what they see in others that they wouldn't have thought about if it hadn't been presented to them. These are just some of, possibly hundreds of, corresponding behaviors resulting in a reaction to insecurity.

People who have come into their own understanding of power within themselves have noticed *when* they are watching the mirror in themselves through others. The psychologists say that we could be more observant of our Selves if we "see that what we don't like in others is what we don't like in ourselves." Some would argue that point and say, "Absolutely not! I would never do something like that to someone!" Of course, pulling certain behaviors would seem ridiculous, yet we could benefit from being the observer. My suggestion to everyone would be to be as aware as you can possibly be without judgment on ANY level. If we had only sacred confidence in our being, we would observe and become more compassionate, creative, factual, independent, happy, peaceful, understanding, non-judgmental… positive. Mostly, we would be *healthy*. The bottom line of truth in health for the soul is this:

How you feel about yourself determines your own physical health. This goes beyond diet and exercise! Of course, diet and exercise are important to the body, but let's not lose sight of that which is sacred unto yourself… your soul.

~ POINTERS FOR HEALING ~

Here are 10 pointers for healing that will help you on a daily basis:

1. Stay in the moment! This is where all power of life exists and creates the way of alignment with Universal Intelligence.
2. *Pay Attention.* You are the only one responsible for your actions, reactions, and non-actions!
3. *Be the Observer.* All of life is based on our perspectives...
4. Be careful in taking life too personally. It was meant to enjoy, not fight.
5. Be honest with yourself at all times.
6. *Listen* with more than your ears. See with more than your eyes. Insights and Truths can be gained through this allowance.
7. *Be aware* of your thoughts, your words and your actions.
8. Quit blame altogether. There has never been a case recorded that anyone has ever healed because they blamed something or someone.
9. Remember that every moment you live you are making a choice. How precious is that?
10. *Be gentle* to yourself. We all are learning how to expand our awareness.
11. Give yourself the space and time necessary to reflect. Beating yourself up won't heal the pain.

Below is a list I've put together that might help you in how to see blockages, on any level, that eventually restrict the flow in any part of the body. Blockages, such as the effects of our insecure actions, restrict the body's potential for healing. This can include blood, nerve, oxygen, and any forward motion toward a goal. These obviously cause dysfunction and discomfort as well. Here are some common themes I've read through performing energy work in others when it comes to conditions in the physical body:

Allergies: Blockages in the stomach and intestines …what are we not digesting?

Alzheimer's: Preferring the old ways over the new. Why can't things just stay the same?

Acne: Disgusted with your own self-image… not sure of what face to show others.

Aching: Craving love so bad, it hurts! (Depending on where the ache is, the language speaks for itself.)

Adrenals: Overused and underpaid! Adrenals are the *fight or flight* receivers and givers of the body for our energy. Also, this can be determined if we are ignoring ourselves in how much we are actually putting out.

Addictions: Lack of self-esteem and not accepting deeper meaning in life. Deliberate ignorance and emotional running.

Anxiety: Fear generated by past experienced not yet released.

Arthritis: Joints are related to this. Joints determine flexibility. How flexible are we willing to be? Not letting go.

Asthma: Fear from past lives, somewhat acknowledged in this life. Feeling alone…not safe.

Bladder: (cystitis) Being pissed off. "But this is all I know!"

Blood Pressure: What pressures stand in our way to freedom?

Bones: Represent past lives and memories stored there. Marrow is the meat of our past.

Bowels: The "outcome" of the day. Pressures either building or releasing.

Breasts: Lack (or not) of love and nurturing for the self. Left side: Am I allowing love into my life? Right side: Am I willing to give love? Am I possibly giving too much??

Bronchitis: Feeling that you can't change a situation happening that is close to your heart. Inner congestion.

Cancer: This brings up inner upset. Deep hurts unresolved. Anger toward self.

Candida: "Can anybody hear me?" Lack of trust. Deep frustrations not recognized.

Carpal Tunnel: "Why can't I make this life work?" It's a form of outward frustration relating to the nerves held deep under the armpit. This is also where we keep our deepest secrets so others can't see them.

Cerebral Palsy: A complex, yet most loving way a person comes in to this world. Loving toward family, and yet in a Spiritual world, not understood by many. When one of our senses leaves us, another gets stronger. In this case, the spirit over the body. CP is the most loving and yet Spiritual condition. Anger and frustration come from "Why don't they understand me?"

Cold Hands and Feet: Not trusting yourself. Believing you may never "live up to...."

Colds: We simply don't catch colds. Colds are mental confusion. Not sure if you should choose one way or another.

Coughs: Not sure how to express your deepest concerns or fears.

Cramps: Not relaxing with the flow of your life. Feeling that there has got to be more!

Depression: Making yourself stay in a situation or feeling that you hate. Depriving yourself happiness because you feel committed.

Dizziness: Scattered thinking. Confusion of the next intent. Sensitive instability.

Edema: Tears not released. Better to cry. Swollen emotions.

Fat: Oversensitivity. Sadness. A need for a way of protection. Where is all this weight coming from?(can also be holding onto others or your own emotions in the body.)

Fatigue: Boredom, resistance, and denying what it takes to move forward. "What's next?"

Fevers: Anger. Burning up inside. Emotions not released.

Fibroids: Questioning if you are loved. Nursing pains from the past.

Flu: Time out. This is your body's way of making yourself slow down.

Gum problems: Not making a decision for yourself and not sticking to it if you did! Be clear, and go for it!

Hands: Represent holding on or letting go.

Hay Fever: Not feeling that you deserve to be happy. A form of self persecution.

Jaws: Coping with life. "How do I do it?"

Insomnia: Fear, guilt, and a feeling that "I just can't control life…"

Itching:	Nerves encountering a situation left unresolved.
Kidneys:	Disappointment. No real support. Feeling unloved. Pissed off.
Lymph problems:	Hiding your inner most feelings. Over sensitivity to an emotional cause. and not dealing with it.
Muscles:	Representing our ability to move in life. How flexible are we?
Nail biting:	Not liking yourself and wondering if you really have anything to offer. Questioning your worth.
Nerves:	Communication with yourself…or Not!
Parkinson's:	Not learning how to give love to the self. Unfulfillment . Overboard for others…obligation.
Pneumonia:	I'm so tired… trying just isn't necessary anymore.
Skeletal:	Past lives unresolved. Deep core cellular memory not yet acknowledged.
Spasms:	Holding onto old thoughts when old thoughts are ready to be let go of.
Sacrum:	Represents what are you sitting on? Let's get to the bottom of the issue.

Teeth: Represents not liking your situation. (Because they are bone, it could be past life pain coming up for release

Ulcers: Not feeling fulfilled. Leaving a hole and causing grief.

Seizures: " I've really had enough and I'm going to show you!"

These are only a few conditions with associated causes. When you begin to realize how this makes sense that the body is our barometer, our communicator, our answer to the recognition necessary to identify what we *haven't* recognized about ourselves, we will begin to pay attention and then understand more of the communication our beautiful body is trying to tell us.

Pain indicates a condition due to an unresolved situation. However, if we do not want to be in constant pain, we must be careful not to allow ourselves to instantly feel fear. The knowledge of pain isn't meant to bring in fear…it's meant to associate something we might be missing in our conscious awareness. If we practice this perception, we will find that knowledge of the human body then becomes our friend. Maybe this is what was meant with the saying, "Be your own best friend!" I accept that one!

~ Something's WRONG, you say? ~

Many people are still under the influence of believing in a concept that pain indicates that something is wrong and we need to see someone to identify the problem. I have seen so many cases of where a client comes in with muscle pain, joint pain, or a diagnosed condition leaving the client immobile or inflexible. There's nothing worse than desiring to be active and knowing that your body doesn't want to follow suit.

In years past, our acceptable trained thought around health was either thinking we were doing something wrong or something could be wrong. As time continues, that is the past. The current trend in energetic medicine is about you, the person behind the driver's seat!

By changing our perception of how our bodies feel, we can actually "hear" a cause if we listen closely enough. This, however, takes quite a bit of discipline and non-attachment to the pain through the mental mind. We can use the other bodies we have to co-create healing within, and it is similar to hypnosis; however, we are conscious of directing an initial confrontation to what is going on that is getting our attention. For example, if your arm is achy and it stems from the shoulder…by putting all of your attention on the pain, you forgot to use the other parts of your make up to help you identify why that shoulder hurts. You could apply it with an emotional cause or a mental cause. You can even say that the Spiritual body is at work nudging you to pay attention to how much you are putting out without the proper balanced energy to continue giving. If we say "The weight of the world is on our shoulders" and then feel we HAVE to keep pushing, eventually, we know the shoulder will give out. The idea here is to recognize that there are reasons for the body to talk to you and become the bio-feedback that you need to understand for your own motives, your desires, and your intentions.

Nothing is random. If it were, then there could possibly be no gravity holding us in place and we could all be floating around. The word _random_ seems to be overused and undefined; therefore, it becomes a cute excuse used for a real situation that is part of our living at the moment we choose on any level.

I've heard so many people tell me that they are clumsy, and that's why they fell. Truthfully, they are going through an insecure time and not feeling real good about themselves at that very moment that they fall. Therefore, not watching your step kicks in and a result happens. "To every action is a reaction," my mentor used to say! Using the saying "Random acts of kindness" is sweet, and at the risk of sounding like Sheldon Cooper in the Big Bang Theory TV series…they aren't random at all! They are intentional in the very second you make the decision to smile at a stranger on the street. Sometimes we will find ourselves walking into something or stubbing the same toe over and over. I found through the read of the body that this isn't random either. It's actually a pressure point on your body needing to be released to either help one of your organs to free up to keep the rhythm and flow going, or it could even clear up sinus congestion!

In today's times, with all the changes actually seeming to be speeding up, our physical bodies are also trying their best to keep up with our subconscious thoughts. However, the subconscious is more and more conscious as we expand our awareness into realizing that we are really in charge on a higher level. That's why the integration of your thoughts and actions are being recognized sooner and you might just prevent a fall or some reaction to a cause…simply by finding that you are taking responsibility for your self-esteem and putting your foot forward!

~ OUR RESPONSIBLE AWARENESS ~

"We are not victims of our genes. We are masters of our genes."
~ *Dr. Bruce Lipton* ~

Way before our fabulous friend, author, and Cellular Biologist, Bruce Lipton came into our lives, I had already seen hundreds of people that were experiencing beliefs of themselves that were not theirs. They had been handed set beliefs on a platter, without ever realizing that they were only that! I am very grateful that the door is opening you to the awareness of the knowledge of Jesus who said, "The truth will set you free."

Our parents only knew what they knew, and the concept of blaming them is absurd as we realize it just isn't their fault for all of the mistakes that we see they made. The problem arises when we see ourselves becoming like them if we didn't feel supported in the first place! It makes sense then that once we witness this or that action, we will catch it and, therefore, break the cycle so as to tell the subconscious that this is bigger than you thought consciously and are now going to reconsider and humble to the fact that you never want to act that way again.

If we can see this to be true, then we need to take it a step further. If you look deeper, you will see that we are learning about heredity through knowledge of quantum physics. We can change our perceptions if we have a desire to shift them. Usually however, you need to be ready for that.

In today's world, we're there. We are fed up with old conditioning that obviously does not work for us anymore. We strive to be independent and confident. How wonderful that is! Now, the hard part of our conditioning is that we were born into a society that told us what to think about our health. Therefore, you go to a doctor and they are going to hand you a form to fill out first thing. The questionnaire is going to ask you if your parents had heart failure, diabetes, high blood pressure, etc. After answering this, you find yourself wondering if you also will have that…which makes the visit to the doc a little scarier. (If you didn't have high blood pressure, you probably might now!) So we were, and still are, being told that a major diagnosis will run in the bloodline, and you too can have this condition that can eventually kill you. At this point, my observation is… if the condition doesn't take you out, surely the medicine will! Either way, it's absolutely important to know that you are definitely not a victim to your family traits unless you have similar personalities that create the condition in the first place. Old belief systems are disempowering to your health at this point. You are responsible to determine how healthy you will be. Will it just be your diet and exercise that you feel takes care of you? Could it possibly be your workouts? (God forbid you skip a day!) These are all fine and dandy for keeping strong, fit and in shape. Yet I remember hearing the news of a doctor in my town that was extremely healthy. He ran every day at lunchtime, and had a big family. One day he went on his usual run and fell over with a massive coronary that killed him in an instant. Shock and rumors traveled throughout the clinic. No one really knew what caused that, yet I suspected the running was too much for the organs in his body. The hiatal muscle crept up higher and higher until his breathing became more shallow, putting too much pressure on the heart itself.

——

Several years ago, a wonderful book hit the shelves called <u>The Hiatal Hernia Syndrome</u>. (I happened to be reading this when this doctor had fallen over with his coronary.) As a Medical Intuitive hands on therapist, I saw cases of a high hiatal way too often. What caught my attention was that many doctors didn't! The book was put out by Davis University in Northern California where years of study went into this. What was profound was that the study showed 99 different diagnoses in relation to the hiatal being too high. It could determine the reason for a pain in the shoulder, a tickle in the throat, all the way to a heart attack. It definitely is significant of heartburn or as they say acid reflux. There are amazing effects of a hiatal muscle that worked its way up into the cavity of the lung, causing a protrusion into the tissue putting pressure on the lungs, heart, and diaphragm. That means circulation, oxygen and the capacity to breathe are all now restricted. What is also true is that most of us have a hiatal that is up there, and fortunately, have not had to endure the horrific results of it turning into a hernia. Yet the effects are still shallow breathing and poor circulation. That in turn prevents oxygen which stops the clarity of thought, and mostly, true relaxation.

If we learn how to properly exhale and shove the little muscle down from right under the xyphoid process in between the rib cage, we would have more circulation, more oxygen, and clearer thinking… along with 99 less possibilities of being incorrectly diagnosed!

The body has many wonderful ways of healing itself. It is in constant homeostasis. We are the ones who throw it off, mostly through a lack of true awareness.

~ LEFT IS RECEIVER, RIGHT IS GIVER ~

Many of my clients have had surgery based on the pain that comes from the low back. The low back is essentially the common place where people are insecure to their own support. The tailbone is about survival. In a person's being if they feel they are not supported, many times the hips will go out of alignment. We all have this from time to time, but a chronic situation is inevitably going to produce a result, as every action has a reaction. In this case, the left hip up can cause pressure eventually in a woman not only in her intestine, but also in her ovary, or her bladder. It's pressure on the front as well as the back. For a man, it can be that he carries his wallet in the left back pocket, causing the left hip to eventually go out after a period of time, which in turn can cause prostrate blockages, urinary dysfunction, and even diverticulitis. After a while, like in any situation, something's gotta give. A doctor doesn't see this. They immediately know that you are in pain, and many times only know to recommend surgery. So many surgeries are incredibly avoidable. Yes, a Chiropractor can get it back in, however, it can go out again and again…good for the Chiropractor, but not so good for you. Knowing what causes this is important. The left hip that is too high is a reaction to the receiving hip saying, "I can't take anymore unsupported action in my life. I refuse to accept it." So it actually blocks the support area by moving up and defending itself. The same goes for the right hip. The right is the giving side, and when the hip goes out on the right, it is usually significant of the energy of saying, "I refuse to give out support anymore to others. So there!"

A diagnosis can only tell us the possibilities of an outcome, but down deep, it can be an incorrect judgment and can definitely cause more pain in the long run. The body will enlighten you as to why it needs to share its opinion, because

---

it is your barometer. Just like if your smoke detector smells smoke. It will set off an alarm to warn you that something is happening and smoke is detected. The body and the area of the body also are those alarms. It will set itself off for you to recognize that it needs your attention. When your dog is hungry, she gives you a look and demands then the dinner that she requests. You wouldn't think twice about not having your dog fed, your car taken care of, or your appliances fixed. Then why do we deny the pain that is the sound off that wants our attention? It's time to see the reasons behind the actions of the body, to which, by all standards of quantum understanding, we are not victims. Today we often hear, "There are no accidents." I support this through all of the body work I have seen. Nothing is random.

~ TAKING YOUR STAND ~

Many years ago, I had a friend who did healing work out of her home. One day she invited me to come to her house and have tea and a chat! Agreeably, I went with glee knowing that when it came to chatting about health, nothing could please me more!

She told me a story of a dear friend of hers that recently had passed of cancer.

It was an amazing and true situation that we all could learn from on every level.

She told it this way;
"One afternoon a beautiful Native American woman went to the doctor for a checkup after finding that she did not feel well. Her doctor did a few tests and came back to inform

her that she had cancer. He proceeded to tell her that she had six months to live. At this point, the woman slapped the doctor right across the face and said to him, "How dare you! Who do you think you are? That is between me and my God. You have no right to tell me or anyone else how long we have to live!" The woman lived 3 more years.

Then one morning she woke up early. She called six of her friends that were very close to her. She asked them to come over to her house as soon as they could. When they arrived she had informed all of them that she was ready to die. Her exact words were, "Today is a good day to die." She gave each of them a hug and blessings. She then laid herself down and crossed her arms comfortably. Quietly, with much dignity and grace, she slowly slipped away. My friend was one of the people that had been at her house that morning. I was honored to be told that story, especially since I was working at the hospital at the time.

Many people go to a doctor and do not ask questions. They feel like they are at the principal's office at school and aren't sure what they are going to be told. Therefore, they usually take what they hear as fact and leave. Sometimes on the way home they wonder why they didn't ask more questions.

Patients who came in for appointments always had their vitals taken by me before the doctor came into the room. Many had high blood pressure. However, when I applied the technique of visualization, their blood pressure had dropped before the doctor came in. I had them visualize with their eyes closed a scene of being in a field of beauty. This could be flowers, grassland, mountainside streams nearby, or even watching fish swim. By the time the doctor came into the room their heart rate had slowed and their minds were calmer. The white coat syndrome was curable in minutes!

It's time to put responsibility back into our health. If we feel comfortable seeing a doctor, at least have the questions you want answered up front. If the doctor cannot answer them you will usually go for a second opinion. I had a client who had pain in his hand and was sent to 3 doctors and all of them had a different diagnosis. One even said he had the onset of diabetes! *What*? Where ever he got that answer was almost as bad as when a doctor tells you it's all in your head. So seeing a physician ought to be like a job interview. This time, however, you are interviewing the physician. This also reminds me of a realtor. If a house that you are looking to buy might have a leaky roof, you would seek out the truth or even look at a different house. This is how it must be if you are to see a doctor. Use your common sense and see if what he tells you feels right. After all, he needs a code, and what he tells you may generally be all he can see from where he sits. Working in the field was wonderful for what I learned, however, one thing I learned was never to be a patient!

4.

~ Language Beyond Words ~

"Solitary trees, if they grow at all, grow strong."
- Sir Winston Churchill

Remember that term I spoke of earlier, "As Above, So Below?" It's been determined that memories make up our very being. If this is true, then it would make sense that we created our own physical body. The way of living a healthy, more vivacious life for ourselves seems to be how we interpret our lives through perceptions and beliefs. More and more, we are recognizing that old belief systems are not necessarily true to our own soul anymore. We have become challenged as these times in our world are shifting and changing. We are actually becoming more expanded as time moves on through our mental and emotional bodies.

So how can this work in the sense of healing old crippling diseases? How do we see and know what is actually occurring in the body when we get diagnosed by a doctor?

First of all, we have to be willing to learn about it. Most people are so accustomed to going to a doctor and being diagnosed and treated; however, many of us have realized that a doctor just may not know why a condition has happened in the first place. Some of them are even willing to admit that! (God bless them!) They treat what they see and are not necessarily going to tell you emotional causes, etc. They simply cannot, and that is not their job. I feel it is unfair to blame an M.D. when we have just as much responsibility, if not more, for our own health as they do to help us locate a problem or give us a diagnosis.

I have been an energy runner all of my life, working to help heal many people including children. I will never forget the little one year old child that came into my office with her mother. Exhausted and drained by her one year old daughter, the woman was desperate for help. She came in for an appointment to see if I could tell *why* her baby was so clingy, extremely fearful and relentlessly angry about her doing anything around the house without her constantly by her side. She also specified that her baby was born with a giant cyst on her left buttocks that the doctors were saying needed to be removed through surgery.

Well, in order for me to really check out this situation, I had to have "permission" of the child! In order to do this, I had to be able to touch the baby somehow without her getting upset. So I had mom sit on the massage table with the child in her lap. The baby was fine with that, as long as she was touching mommy! So as I observed this behavior further, I realized that this little blonde baby would appreciate it if I tried to give her a crystal out of my collection on the shelf. I asked her which one she wanted. She pointed to a colorful quartz. I gave it to her and watched her as she slightly smiled. As she was observing it, I sneaked my left (receiver) hand on her back very gently. It was OK by her. Then, still sitting on Moms lap, I went down a little further on top of the diaper to see if I could feel (intuitively) the energy of the cyst her mother had told me about. Suddenly, my gut began to contract, and the grief that purged from this area had me crying very hard as silently as I could because I didn't want her to get worried or upset. I endured this massive amount of grief as I wondered how in God's name this could be so strong in a one year old baby. I made myself look through the grief into the cause…which was not easy. I began to see her in the womb at five months old. There was another baby there. Then that one was gone.

I looked up at the mother and asked her a question. "Was this child a twin?" Yes, she was. The twin had died in utero at five months. In the meantime, this baby continued growing and waiting for labor.

This little one year old girl would have been the first born. As I saw the image, the emotion also translated into what I was feeling and seeing. Therefore, in utero, the infants were joined at the buttocks. As the live baby continued to grow, the loss of her sister was transferring to her. She remained clear that she would carry her sister with her by manifesting a physical remembrance in her own body. The cyst was the memory of her sister, and if the doctors would have removed this cyst, the possibility of this baby living would be slim to none. (I find the correlation interesting that the vibration of the word *cyst* and *sister* are very prevalent here)

Separating a cyst of this magnitude would have been devastating for everyone.

Once this energetic knowledge became clear to me, I was able to counteract it with recognition and accepting the emotion that went along with it. This alleviated the child's pain as I took it on.

I continued looking at the situation a little longer, and the baby was still infatuated with the crystal, thank God! I saw that this little girl was very intelligent. The color that fit into her self-confidence was purple. So I told the mom that she needed to buy her a dress right away that was purple with a big yellow flower. If she could find one like that, it would help bring her daughter into her own world and life would ease up for both of them.

One week later, she came back to be re-checked. The mother walked down the hallway to my treatment room, however, the little girl was lagging behind her, not clinging to her. As I laid eyes on the baby, I was shocked. She was wearing a purple dress with a big yellow flower on it. I asked the mom where she got it. She told me, and said, "Guess who picked it out?" Wow! The baby found it. Not only did the little girl quietly come into the room on her own, she was holding a <u>Pat the Bunny</u> book and comfortably plopped herself down to look at it. We all were happy with big smiles…and Mom finally was able to rest.

Stories like this one have been very common in my 29 years of energy healing.

Now, by taking a step further we can begin to energetically identify the language our body gives us through physical expression.

Here is a simple list of how the body speaks:

Arms: What are you carrying and who?

Armpits: Storage unit of what we don't want anyone to see. (emotional)

Breasts: Nurturing the Self. (or lack of)

Back: Relates to Stress, mostly questioning life in relation to support. (who supports us or do they?) Lessons on supporting ourself through love.

Bladder: Emotional resistance to life. Letting go can be so very hard to do.

Calves: Moving forward. Not dealing with past issues or patterns.

Colon: Going with or not in the "flow" of life. Not accepting change.

Eyes: How do you see life? Is it correct to your True Self?

Feet: How we walk in this world. In which direction are we walking?

Heart: Not listening to our *true* self through our feelings.

Hips: General support. When they slip out, it generally relates to an imbalance to how you are relating to life. Feeling the lack of love and support.

Joints: Flexibility to or in your situations…

Kidneys: Holding on to resentment or anger. Feeling pissed off.

Knees: Seeing life as unsupported. Inside knee is community, job, friends

Liver: Old past hurts or current hurts not being released.

Neck: Flexibility or unwillingness to be flexible. Willingness to see different sides of a situation

Nerves: Sensitivity towards a situation not acknowledged.

Ovaries:	Very sensitive past issues about creativity. Guilt stored.
Sinus:	Confusion. Letting go on a mental level.
Shoulders:	Carrying the weight for yourself or others.
Stomach:	Carries recognition of the digestion of real life.
Swollen Conditions:	Tears unshed.

Now, not all parts of the body are mentioned, and that is because I am only giving you a summary.

The body speaks for itself. Sometimes it's a little more complicated. It depends on what, when, and how these conditions were revealed in the "As above" to create the "So below." For example, if we carry a thought that because our mother died of breast cancer, we may feel the energy of that in our breast, eventually causing the fear that then creates the condition. Guilt for staying alive after our parent died can also cause us to deteriorate.

The body only responds to us. That is what it knows how to do. None of us are victims to a mystery. There is no such thing. The physical body has a good reason for everything it encounters. It's up to us to notice how it recognizes and delivers.

~ THE CONNECTION ~

We need to BEGIN with the simple understanding that our body is our vehicle, and just like a car, needs to be maintained, cleaned up, tuned up, and fixed up when repairs are needed. (And just because it has high miles, it can still keep running just fine as long as we take care of it.) Therefore, the body parts are meant for clarity and precision in doing their job. Not only do the organs have a purpose, but so do the limbs, the trunk, feet and hands, etc. They all represent meaning for us to comprehend. Energetically, they all have a metaphoric logic, if you will, to identify their meaning for you.

Even though some of these parts may seem self-explanatory, such as hands are about holding on or letting go and feet are for taking us where we are going, they also have connected reasons to the rest of the body.

The head is a good place to begin. Not only does it hold our senses, but it connects to the rest of the body through the spine, nerves, and directs blood flow and feeds our stomach, and the brain tells us everything beyond our wildest dreams! However, the energetic part of us intends to teach us that we are also led by the spiritual side within to hear and listen beyond our ears, see beyond our eyes, know when a situation "smells fishy". This is what draws us to intuition. The human being, no matter what you've heard, is not stupid by any means. Logically, the physical body cannot be deemed as stupid or incompetent in any way, shape or form. It knows exactly what it's doing, and, at the risk of being redundant, only listens to our perceptions and beliefs which then feeds the cells and becomes the physical body....as above, so below. So why do we feel we cannot change a situation within our body?

70

As an energy healer, I remember telling clients even back in the 70's that we are riddled with insecurities, which then causes a Ricochet effect in the physical body. I have seen over 200 of these nasty critters lurking in the systems of the most wonderful hearted people and have counseled and treated the body through the energy read of the insecurity itself. This then is what our body relates to, hears, and eases into a calmer state. True recognition and confrontation on an energetic level sets you free. When you hear it from someone, whether it be an energy healer or your best friend, it becomes bio-feedback through sound and understanding. It takes that recognition to produce a positive result just as when Alcoholics Anonymous says that you first have to recognize you have a problem.

Life IS fair in the physical body because it is what we chose at higher levels to experience in order to learn this time around. The best part is that we can change it right here and now. It simply isn't bad or good. It is our interpretation of why we are judging ourselves that causes the insecurity in the first place. Here lies the problem. On some level, we have become our own worst enemy, subconsciously to some degree.

My good friend asked me one time what caused Fibromyalgia. When I told her the answer of the energetic read, she responded with, "I think if I had that I'd hit you!" Of course, my response was, "Are you sure you don't have it?" Then I smiled and let that one go.

Any dis-ease we have that has created a form of pain or stress in our body has to come from our world in which we perceive it even if we find that we wake up in the morning with a sore shoulder, and we didn't even work out the day before. Pain just doesn't show one day and release the next by accident. The body can't help but memorize an experience. For example, let's say you are in a car accident. Sudden trauma occurs to the neck. This would be called whiplash.

The body's reaction to this whiplash would be instant trauma, or shock. On some level, the body stores the memory of this like a computer hard drive. Depending on who you are and your idea of this accident, this pain may take a long time to heal. The blood that comes to the tissues during this trauma can cause edema and definitely make you feel stiff and not turn your head very easily. Let's say two years pass. You didn't receive any treatment for it. Your neck is still tight. You are living with it in every way. Now let's say you DID get treatment! You went to an awesome chiropractor. Pain was minimal and your neck wasn't so stiff anymore. Then you went to work one day and you were told that you had a new boss. This boss and you clashed. Your feeling was

1. Shock that you weren't told this was going to happen...
2. You knew you weren't going to get along very well...
3. Now you're worried if you are going to keep your job!

Suddenly you are faced with a situation to which the body resonates ....TRAUMA. Lo and behold, the neck starts to hurt and then you have lack of range of motion, and God forbid you have to take time off time to see a doctor!

This is a type of etheric biofeedback that is happening beyond your control. In a case like this, it's important to consider that you CAN shift this, and you must if you want to go on living without the idea that all sudden circumstances lead to pain from an old accident. It always amazes me how many people come up with some reason on their own to identify why they are in pain...what must have happened that the logical mind wants to believe so as to avoid the inevitable... the truth.

Of course, in spiritual understandings, even the car accident taught you something. It's hard to live life thinking we create our own reality and then have something like a car accident! Whose fault was that? If we could just remember that blame doesn't serve anyone, and that whatever we attract, even as kids, is a part of the life we chose. We love to hear positive speakers, but do we really listen to them? Do we live what we heard, or do we say, "Yea, they were good…. but I'll never remember it all!" Do we even refer to our notes that we took after one month?

What did we get from the phrase "The Law of Attraction"? Is there more to this phrase in life, or were we just hoping we'd get rich from it?

There truly are NO accidents. In every single situation, we learn. If we didn't learn that we were taught to become better for obvious reasons, then why be living? Lessons are life, and life is lessons. In every moment, we own our choice. We can change it any time we want to. Hence, we have the term PERCEPTION.

~ BECOMING THE OBSERVER ~

When I was 7, I was sitting in our living room doing what a kid does. I was observing what it was like to close one eye and open the other, and then quickly switch it by opening the other and closing the other. At this point, I was watching a change in how I saw what was in front of me. My mom watched me doing this and said, "Now what are you doing?" I told her, "I'm watching different worlds out of each eye."

Isn't it funny how we term our perceptions on how we view what we see?

If you've heard the term *Observer* before, more than likely you've studied metaphysics for a long time or even found that as time went on in your life, you might have wanted to be someone else. Many kids experience that feeling when they're young…wanting what others have because they don't like something about their own life.

Believe it or not, this is usually how the ability to become the observer occurs at a very young age. It takes something meaningful to pull a child out of their surroundings on any level (emotionally or mentally) so they don't get locked into only *their* world. Same occurs when a child has an imaginary friend. They seem to be just fine pouring a cup of tea for the party that isn't visible… we aren't. Many parents would like to discount that friend immediately and prefers to bring the child back to reality. I'm sure there are counselors who would disagree with me; however, I had an imaginary friend but he wasn't imaginary to me at all. I spoke with him, laughed with him, and even thought he would send me messages at night when I was sleeping. I won a spelling contest in 1st grade and knew it was he who whispered the letters to me. When I wrote poetry for my mother at a very young age, it was he who helped bring in the words to finish the masterpiece.

Somehow, my mom knew something was up because, as she so often had said, "You're such a weird kid!" One day we were going through some old boxes in the garage, and she brought out a nickel wrapped in tissue paper. When she began to unwrap it, a tear came to her eye. I noticed how sad this made her, and then she told me this was a nickel she saved that my brother, two years older, had swallowed. Then she brought out a lock of his hair which was so blonde, it shocked me. We were living in LA at the time, and Danny had died when I was six months old. He was the first heart transplant patient at the age of three to receive a new heart. His heart was very deformed, very spongy, and just couldn't pump well. So the doctors in 1958 decided to try this surgery on a child. There was one other boy scheduled for the same procedure, and he lived through his surgery. Danny, however, did not. He was the 5th in our family, and I was the 6th and the last.

My mother told me of his heart that day in the garage, and needless to say, I shouted out, "So that's my friends name… Danny!"

I don't remember her exact reaction, except it was *pretty quiet* around the house for a while after that.

I like to speak of being an observer in life. It helps tremendously with identifying what you *don't* want! When our siblings got in trouble, we saw their actions and why they got a spanking. We knew to NOT do what they did, and this is a form of being an observer. When we know as adults when to keep our mouths closed because our coworkers won't like the remarks we want so badly to make, we are the observer in that situation. When you care about others and feel their concerns, or your baby cries and you sense he's hungry. Your mother calls yelling at you, and somehow you realize it's not you she's yelling at, at all…it's the fact she broke her favorite vase trying to arrange it for a dinner party that night. These are examples of being the observer in life to the nearest and dearest to you. If we take everything too personally, it becomes selfishness on our part and we negate a compassion that sits waiting for us to observe.

When we reach a point in life, for example a midlife crisis, and we are aware that we might be feeling sorry for ourselves, we listen internally and suddenly realize "How will I choose to react to this emotion?" *That's* being the observer. Being the observer is basically a keen sense of awareness that you catch through yourself and through others. It's where you see life from a small distance, not to ignore it or even to deny it. It's a way to interpret a fact at that moment… and just be the witness. You are witnessing life as an observer.

One of the reasons this is a way of life that works wonderfully is because you can see the big picture from here. It's where the mind takes you away from the ego perspective and shows you an alternative to emotion. It gives you a fact instead of an attached emotion.

~ ATTACHMENT vs. DETACHMENT ~

When you hear the word *attachment* what could be the first thing you think? You might consider it to be a comforting thought. Some wonder if it's good or bad. Others will tell you "That's my problem...I attach to everything!" Heck, we can even attach to attachment!

The truth I found in reading energy is this... it is neither good nor bad. These concepts do not exist in the higher realms of consciousness. We made decisions to judge what we consider good or bad a long time ago, but it really narrows down to perceptions and opinions of our actions and reactions. Perception is the true reality of our world. Attachment then is when we have made the decision to connect in a form where the ego lives.

A client many years ago asked me to read the energy of her sister.

I had to explain to her that by Universal Law, it was not respectful or even allowed for me to read someone else's stuff without their consent.

However, what I could do for her, the client, was to help her heal herself and that in turn would free her up from the worry and fear that she had around her sister and her issues. I explained that we could help ease her concern that her sister might die. She understood, but then said to me, "So I'm not helping my sister by worrying about her, am I?" The sad truth was no, she wasn't helping anything. She realized after recognizing her fears that it was only transferring into the weakness of her sister.

This was a very important moment of truth for her. About a week later, I received a phone call from her. She called to tell me that her sister was now getting stronger and even their conversations were better! There was even laughter instead of dread.

We confuse attachment with loving. Attaching is a principle we use to help us feel like we have something close to our hearts, when in reality, the closeness we feel can never really expand into a life generated by love if we deem it necessary to hold on through attachment. It eventually becomes conditional and then we may lose instead of gain.

In the same way, due to our learning as children, we became attached to what we thought we *should* do...either for our parents, our peers, or even God. In the meantime, we forgot to see through the eyes of the moment and experience our feelings from a clearer perspective, rather than thinking we had to have an attached outcome. This is where we are today. The children of our time are much more aware that they live completely and honestly in the moment. They state how they feel, what they see, and where they perceive truth to be. Nothing can stop these kids from this enormous joy within themselves, unless they feel stifled by an attachment of duty.

In order for us to be free thinkers and feelers, we must realize that independence is crucial, yet know that oneness is a natural state of being. We can have a multitude of expansive communities of people who have a keen sense of this loving desire to work as a unit. However, for us to exist well and be well in this world, this must come from individual acceptance within each person. Then the community works as a team, and not under the thumb of some democracy telling us how to do it.

If we continue to live by the standards of others' decisions for us, we are doomed to misunderstand the true concepts of living. We do not have arranged marriages anymore for the simple reason that it wasn't our decision in the first place! Heck, I can hardly watch the movie "Fiddler on the Roof" anymore just for that reason alone... however, that doesn't take away the love I have and carry for that sweet father played by Topol. You've just got to love his passion for his daughter's happiness!

Inside our bodies, the language tells me that it does not desire confusion. More than likely, that alone can set off many dysfunctional patterns that lead to illness. Today, so many people are experiencing this state of living through chaos. This is affecting our immune system because it is related to the nervous system, and each of them are hyper-extending themselves through fear as releases begin to come up and come out. If we understand that we can no longer hold onto the attachments of the past and have the courage to see this, then we will understand that the body will be releasing *through* chaos, as our world is also doing. Therefore, it is not a bad thing that this is occurring. It is a blessing so that truth can find its way in through these cracks of acceptance and then we have light to lead us in the next step of our evolutionary process. This is what we call ENLIGHTENMENT and is ultimately where this world is heading, sooner or later.

We are not necessarily detaching, we are becoming more aligned to the oneness aspect of our true self. Our health is related to this configuration as oneness continues to become clearer within ourselves.

5.

You and Your Body...
A Cosmic Marriage

"If so much energy is in one beam of light, think of how much power one human has in one thought. All beings have the capacity to heal themselves." -The Movie; K-Pax

"As Above, So Below"

If you've never heard the term "As above, so below," it's a term I like to use to identify how energy works with the human body. Most people have heard by now, thanks to movies like, "What the Bleep Do We Know?" that like attracts like, and your thoughts are things. Many authors today are using this quantum expression to get the word out on The Law of Attraction.

In the energetic readings I've done on the human body for over 25 years, I learned that "as above, so below" holds true to all experiences and thoughts, either in the past, the present or even the future! "As above" includes your mental body, your emotional body, and your Spiritual subconscious. The "so below" portion is our physical body. Your body is its own entity, mimicking your every thought, every experience and every situation in a decision you've made or a feeling you had. The kicker is that our body knows us better than anyone ever could!! It heard you. It hears your inner most secrets and your little white lies. It hears the excitement of a new relationship and the grieving of a death…one that even occurred 40 years prior. There's nothing the body doesn't know about you. It even taps into your subconscious mind and pays attention!

The term "As Above, So Below" is important to consider when talking about the marriage of you and your body. Many authors and teachers have shared their knowledge about the Spiritual body, the mental body, and the emotional, causal and etheric bodies. We have learned about how our thoughts are things and that we create our own reality. Rarely, however, have I heard very many people talk about how the cellular memory process works in the physical form when it comes to bodywork and the releasing of this.

In the experiences of my work, I have definitely come to the conclusion that _all pain is energy_. All parts of the body have something to say. It's like they all have their reason for being where they are and why they act and react to aches, pains, and sometimes becoming much more. Therefore, conditions (or as some people call "diagnosis") happen for reasons that are not seen or detected by an MRI.

As like the Universe, energy in our bodies doesn't know the difference between right or wrong…it just knows how to respond to an "intent." Our intent is our desire. The heart picks this feeling up and immediately transports it to the nearest port that has similar cell patterns that it can identify with. That port can be under the armpit, (that's where people store their deepest emotions that they don't want others to know about) or, for another example, the thigh. That would indicate the support (or lack of) in you of moving forward.

It can be anywhere, on any pressure point, or even down the spine. One woman I had seen was an actress, and her life was depicted through the apex of each vertebrae! Honestly, from the top of the spine (the atlo-axis) to the tailbone, she told her own story. I read from the time she was a 17 year old looking for work, then a boyfriend/ marriage, then her career, a divorce, the job, and finally, depression that had set in the tailbone!! Whew! All this just in her spine! That didn't include the rest of the muscle memory.... This lovely lady decided to hang on to all of her feelings, and literally bury them in bone. People might do this because they don't want to forget their experiences, and have decided to hold on to them. Even though we might think that's a hard way to live, for her, it was the way she chose to learn spiritually... bone always represents past lives, or past living. People store their emotions, mental ideas and wishes, and even their Spiritual concepts directly in certain areas of their physical form. These areas can be in any muscle, leg, arm, etc. that depends on where a trauma has hit or a place in the body that recognizes intensity. If a runner who has run for many years develops more leg cramps, would this be due to the idea that the person is not getting the fluids necessary? Maybe it's a Chemical shift in the body? Maybe it's that he is just lacking potassium? Or could it possibly be that, in fact, the person has decided to "stop running" from life and decided to get involved? Leg pain is usually about moving forward. Left side is receiving... on everyone. Right side is giving. If the runner begins to get heavy leg cramps on the right leg, the read might be that she /he is giving out too much from themselves and not paying enough attention to the need inside. Moving forward, then, has been ignored, and has given the body the idea that "enough is enough!" The person is then ready to stop running so much and get on with life from a different perspective.

~ LISTENING TO THE BODY~

The body loves when we hear it speaking.

I remember when I was five years old, my mother had lain down on the couch after 10 hours of working. She had turned on the television to relax. I sat down next to her and, even then, asked her if I could rub her feet. The look on her face was precious! "Of course!" she exclaimed... then came the best foot rub ever, so I thought! She did the cutest thing as I started rubbing her foot. She began to wiggle the one that wasn't receiving the rub at that time and acted like that foot could talk. Her expression was priceless when she began talking with a wiggle in her foot, saying, "What about me? Don't forget me!" So I put the foot down I was working on and rubbed the foot that was complaining. Within two minutes, she began doing the same thing with the other foot, then the other one. Even though I was feeling like her feet were selfish and wanted me all to themselves, I learned at that time the body actually DOES talk...even though my mom spoke for hers!

Little did I know back then, at five years old, I would be doing this for a living one day, and learned from my mother about body talk. It will tell you when it wants attention for sure!

We have been told by science that we shed our cells on a regular basis, and every 11 weeks we have a new liver, after six weeks, we get new kidneys, and after a few months, we are apt to have built naturally a whole new body! If this is the

82

case, then why do we have chronic pain and continue to hurt, even at the risk of getting worse?

Every cell in your body has memory. Author and Cell Biologist, Bruce Lipton, has told us that we have five trillion cells in our body acting as a community. They either get along or work things out or they have environmental "debt", so to speak, and cannot replenish themselves fast enough to heal, due to the beliefs and the power of our thoughts on being a victim.

Our bodies are storage units, basically, and have a lot of room for more. *Just because we shed the cells doesn't mean we shed the emotion inside.* We carry this information like we're a computer. We keep it in the archives, and then we can pull on it at any time we recognize that we are in a position to use it! For example, let's say when you were very little, your father made a comment jokingly that you made dry brownies when baking with your mother for the first time. You were excited at first to see that your dad was going to get a brownie! To a kid, this is a big deal, right? Then he makes a comment, even jokingly, and it crushed you. You didn't respond, but inside, you felt you had horribly failed as a baker!

So when you are an adult, you go to make dinner for a mate, someone you want to do something nice for... do you think that old memory of your father's comment has left the body? I doubt it. Somewhere in there, you will be ready if your partner doesn't like what you've done for them. Chances are, you might even feel defensive before anything can even be said. Expectations can arise that no matter how good you think you've made it, it won't turn out well. You might also think that you're a lousy cook and shouldn't even attempt to *try* to cook. But somewhere you will carry this memory until you release it and confront it. This, in a sense, is biofeedback to the cells. Emotions are number one with this body of ours, and believe me, it carries hurts, disappointments, trauma, and a lack of self esteem (insecurities) more than any other emotion. This is because the memory was harsh…the feelings of being accepted or not are huge within us. Other emotions are tied in as well, but not as strongly as the harder ones. Reading certain people's muscle memory is like watching the evening news! Each person is so unique, and what they choose to carry, to remember, is what's important for their health later on! The emotional body can create our physical template. Illness can certainly be attributed to our emotions, even before the mental body has a chance to interrupt. The immune system is the most sensitive for holding deep emotions and not recognizing them. Lymphatic action can result in confused states because we are doing what we "thought" we were supposed to be doing in life, either pleasing others too much, but maybe on some other level that we weren't catching, we were angry. Something like this can result in Lymphoma in a very sensitive system. Fevers are unexpressed hatred or deep anger. When we feel we need to live up to someone else's expectations, or even our own sometimes, it can develop into a serious auto-immune condition.

So in conclusion to your health, it's "how" a person interprets an experience that can cause a disruption in the flow of life that in turn can cause a condition in the body called illness.

Years ago, I had a client come in who had a condition called "scleroderma." This is an auto-immune dysfunction of a very interesting kind. My experience with this read was that, no matter what this person had told me in regards to the medical diagnosis and explanation, (which they have not found a cure for) I saw that his body was closing in on itself.

It was like seeing him being put in between two walls that were both closing in on him. Eventually, the tight skin was going to get tighter, the chest would get more closed in, and the heart would eventually be squeezed. Yes, this is known as fatal.

He had heard of energy treatments and decided to try one with me out of curiosity. (By the way, the statistics for a condition like this are more common to hit women over 40, *not* men at the age of 28. So it was highly unusual to begin with.)

The young man had come in with a slight attitude that didn't seem to me to fit his kind behavior the day I made his appointment. He seemed so sweet, yet there was this edge… he got on my table, and as I explained that energy work could change certain responses in the body, he acted rather surprised. After a few minutes, we began. His girlfriend was in the room with us, and was an absolute doll. She wanted to help, so as his partner, I had her hold his feet while I continued. He shouted out, "What is she doing holding onto my feet when I'm paying you?" I continued anyway, and then explained that partners who want to contribute can help in the process because they care. His response was rough, and so I realized I had to tell him if he kept up this attitude, he'd have to leave. This startled him enough to get him to relax. I asked him, "Do you want to know the reason for your illness from what I'm reading in the energy?" Of course he did. I told him if he continued to be like his father, talk like him, etc, he would not heal. I explained to him that his body was taking on his father's energy so much that his own body was resisting it and causing an inner battle. He responded strongly once more by saying, "How do you know anything about my father?" I said, "You did come to an energy healer, did you not?"

I asked him when was the last time he'd played an instrument?(hard to do when your fingers won't bend). He said it long time, but he missed it. After he recognized that he had taken on large doses of his dad's world, his body heard the news and released it. At one point, I had to use crystals as a laser over his stomach to help release the stronghold in the aura.... At that point, he gave out a scream and then cried. His girlfriend did the same, and of course, I couldn't resist tears as well.

He came back in once a week for six weeks, then he went to the Health Food store to get cell salts (bio-constituents of the tissue used to replace the minerals, etc. that we have lost or used up) and after six weeks, he went back to have the test done to find out where the dis-ease was on the charts or a scale. If you are at zero, you get the news that you are in remission. If you hit 50, you're dead. When he first came in he was at 27. After six weeks, he was at two.

Wouldn't it have been nice if the physician would have asked him if he'd done something different? With no known cure, I think this would have been a very good question!

~ THE EMOTIONAL BODY ~

Our emotions are usually the #1 trigger in how we perceive ourselves. They are what carry the thoughts of ourselves, and they certainly can be harmful if we don't rise above them. However, to deny our real feelings at the time is withholding information to the heart itself, and that eventually will bite you back one way or another. That behavior resonates to a blockage, and then can create one quickly. This alone is what causes a heart attack. After many years of this behavior, we can die from ignorance and

----

denial. So many people have put a callus around their hearts so as to *not* be hurt.

If we didn't have our emotional body, we would not even know what love was. Some still don't; however, the emotional body is what we are mostly about. We simply cannot know who we are if we do not learn from our experiences and our lessons. Actually this can really help when you go through something with this in mind. It makes the pill go down easier, and then you can be much gentler with yourself in the process.

In the 1990 edition of the book entitled, <u>Bringers of the Dawn</u> by Barbara Marciniak, she describes through channeling that emotions are the conductor and the connector to our soul. It is why we came back to Earth in order to understand actions and reactions of people and then to rise above their insecurities until we act out of compassion. (My mentor used to say, "You don't spank a baby for pooping his pants!") This leads you to a greater perspective of life as you realize that judgment has no place in life whatsoever. The lack of judgment is what creates Oneness within us all. The emotional body makes the most important decisions for you in your life. It is directly related to the heart. Remember when I said earlier that pain is energy? It truly is on many levels, mostly due to emotions and interpretations from our own perceptions and/ or insecurity. As we learn to let go of painful words, or painful actions of another, realizing we had a part in it or it would not have happened to us in the first place, the pain eases and we no longer have to depend on an inflammatory (tears unshed) drug or a pain reliever to go on. As Don Miguel gently states in his book <u>The Four Agreements</u>, do not take things personally. (What a gift we have in realizing this is very important, yet also courageous… just as long as we do not try to get revenge!)

~ THE MENTAL BODY ~

In the mental body of our consciousness, we consider the mind to be our decision maker. Do we not consider this to be the job of the mental mind? Isn't that what we were given a brain for…to think? Just like in the Wizard of Oz, the Scarecrow was so proud to know he had been given a brain from the Wizard. Now he could think and be smart, when really, through the whole movie, he was already making decisions out of necessity and survival. We do too, no matter what our IQ says. My dear friend and business partner, John Jay Harper, was a scientist for the Dept. of Defense in the US Army and also was a visionary. The day before he passed away, he made a comment on the radio during an interview. He said, "The scientist in me has to die so the mystic can be reborn." Ironically, he was gone four days later.

Both John and I would discuss the mental body and its pros and cons. It was important to put concepts, equations, and ideas together to come up with a scenario that we could see from the viewpoint of science on where our world was going in 2012 and beyond… until we spoke of the fear it might cause in people and then realized the counter-productiveness in general. If people could change their concepts, perceptions, equations, and ideas of their lives, on a larger scale, this would change the world and possibly prevent the catastrophic conclusion that seemed so grim in the first place.

The mental mind conceives of facts and belief systems. If we bought into religion or any form of idea that refused to shift within us, this could not only stifle the process of growth in a true quantum Universe, as it could also cause a brain tumor, aneurism, stroke, Parkinson's , dementia, and even attract a coma. I mentioned my client with Scleroderma, and if he had stayed in the mindset of his fathers' thinking, this sensitive man could have died of a self-induced auto-immune dysfunction very shortly. So the mental mind has many forms to it. Positively within us on a whole, it can also stimulate emotions by allowing them. It can sense the creative nature of the soul, search out talents and adventures, and make decisions based on logic, not panic. It also can adapt quickly as a humble employer of the heart. The choice is ours with the perceptions we make. When the mental mind harmonizes with the emotional body, our intuition turns into knowledge and trust. We react to circumstances based on the feeling in order to make the decisions we must make. All of this can happen with the proper sense of agreement between the two.

Today it would definitely behoove us to allow these two to become one, since in 2012, our 5th dimension is all about unconditional love and open hearted awareness.

~ THE SPIRITUAL BODY ~

Today more than ever before in history, our spiritual body must be understood for the betterment of the whole. This is, in retrospect, what makes us or breaks us. We cannot deny that we are one unit, living and breathing as we think and feel, so how does the Spiritual body play a part in this whole thing? Does it mean the religion we believe and follow? Could it mean our understanding of God?

Truthfully speaking, in my work as a reader, it is none of that. Our spiritual body is the one within that acts and reacts to life. It's the observer, the over-soul that brings in the desires, the questions, the choices, etc. This is our subconscious. Those who realize that life never dies and that we have been here before in other lifetimes ultimately can understand that this life is a continuation of the prior ones giving us another chance at making our life better. The spiritual body's total intent is to get us to oneness, since there is no separation in the larger picture anyway. It is a journey to be well recognized. For it is in the recognition that we collide awareness with truth, developing a big bang prospect and eventually bringing in a freedom of joy, bliss, gratitude, etc. If we see it this way for a moment, we will realize that together we are more powerful, especially from the lessons learned.

When I began working as an energy runner in my early days, I had noticed that when working on babies, there was so much more than what we see in a small child. The soul of a child is huge, and in her/his own way, fills a room with his/her "bigness." If one cannot talk or seem aware, he is that much more capable of actually living the spirit within before any conditioning takes place. Clients I've had with cerebral palsy, or even multiple sclerosis, have these spirits that determine their life, as limited as we perceive it. They feel more of everything around them due to a lack of body function. It is like when we lose one of our 5 senses, the others become stronger. This is what happens to clients I've seen with CP or MS. Their spirits are more apt to define their world through energy and see for others a better way of living per say.

On the deathbed of a loved one, we see them slipping away in front of our eyes, yet what we don't see are the days before they die, when the soul's energy permeates the room even when they sleep. Their spiritual body is awakening to its own truth until their need to be here is no more.

As time continues in this dimension of awareness to which we are awaking, we are in our own way expanding as we gain depth in our wisdom, allowance, and humility. Humility is not a weak behavior as we might have thought several years ago. Instead, it is a form of release in feeling that we know so much and open ourselves to more possibilities. It is the opposite of ego. Therefore, our depth perception is increasing and our reality is changing.

The spiritual body will not only guide us to more intuitive coaching, but we are also more capable of seeing the "magic of life" almost as if we have someone watching out for us. We must remember as Humanity, this is the most volatile time in history for us to be able to correlate our ideas, our concepts, and our knowledge and help each other in creating decisions based on the best for the whole. This is done through individual acceptance of our emotional and mental mind to bring in the balance of the whole person, then the whole world. This is what true health is, and where I see each of us going. When the mind and body are aligned to each other, we call this the state of *being*.

6.

~ Illusion to Illumination ~

"If we can remember that fear is the ultimate illusion, then we will ultimately be much clearer in being ourselves." - Mona Delfino~

I love the fact that there have been so many wonderful books out recently which talk about the illusions that we have created in order to feel safe as depicted in books such as "Biology of Belief" by Bruce Lipton, or "Fractal Time" by Gregg Braden. These "science to spirit" kinds of guys have concepts backed by science as fact, which has many people listening today. Isn't it interesting that even 10 years ago, we wouldn't have been able to identify theory over truth? When the movie "Contact" came out with Jodi Foster, it hit the charts. Why? Because it showed that when faced with sight of the Galaxy, unknown to many even at that time, Jodi Foster's character had been so enlightened by what she was observing, that she commented, "I had no idea" with monstrous eyes and a look of amazement to depict her sense of shock.

Living on this planet, we know on some level that life is spoken of as an illusion because we can change it with the way we see our own explanations. Let's take time for example. We set our clocks to the correct time, run our lives by the time, and wonder when we are running OUT of time!! If you see from the idea of Sacred Sight, you can identify that time is definitely an illusion. We set up these standards in order for a communication to occur as to "keep track." If you can see it from a different perspective, you will notice that time doesn't really exist. We created it. It's a lot like money... the idea always remains outside of our true reality. We have placed so much importance on these limited confinements based as reality that we constrict ourselves to them, and judge ourselves because of them. What a circus when you stop and think about it. When you hear phrases like "We're on Indian time" or "Hawaiian time", you know you won't be "on time!" I have found for several years if you listen with your inner abilities, you will wake up when you want to, know when it's time to eat, and trust your inner clock. A friend of mine who decided last minute to ask me to go to a movie never had the desire to actually find out "when" it was playing, and would always seem to call me at that "right" time! I was amazed every time with his ability to know when to tune in and not be concerned as to weather or not we would be late.

When my mentor would ask me to come to her house, I would say," Sure! I'll be there around 4 or so". She would politely say, "Don't tell me what time you will be here because if you aren't here at that time, I'll be worried. Just get here in the afternoon."

Illusion basically is creating something out of either what other people say or it can also be what we buy into from the television, and not knowing for sure if what we are hearing is correct within our consciousness. Illusion doesn't know depth of self, and certainly holds us back from knowing the depth within others. We can make up or say anything we want, but that doesn't make it the best for our growth and understanding. Illusion doesn't know how to alert us to a sense of urgency inside of us. It keeps us superficial in a world of outside influences...and in hopes that we are continuously "doing the right thing," or "making right choices"… even that is an illusion. For many of the illnesses today are created out of this kind of thinking. I guess you could say that both words start with the word, "ill." Therefore, if we become more conscious today of what we are buying form the media, conversations, group meetings, co-workers, etc., you can begin to be your own witness in observing a greater opportunity to see clearer for yourself, not for the sake of pleasing anyone else. What freedom we have in knowing that we can trust our own intelligence and refer to our own destiny as "ours" to be grateful for. This way of looking at your life will help in confronting the old patterns that no longer serve you, or anyone else around you. Health is created from depth of soul centered thinking and living. Sacred Sight has us feel the moment in order to react appropriately for our inner selves. When we come from this place, there is no guilt, no denial, no need for judgment, and a sense of knowing….leading us to *illumination.*

Illumination is seeing clearly from an expansive perspective. I love the word, ILLUMINATION. You don't have to take a class in it. You just learn by experience that wisdom *is* illumination. The deeper you go, the more expansive you get. In the movie, "What the Bleep Do You Know", the question used many times is, "How far down the rabbit hole do you want to go?" That leads us into quantum physics and quantum awareness, but for now we'll stick with these simpler concepts.

You know, something I have observed for years in my work is when I'm in a room of someone who is dying. I have had clients on their death beds knowing that they "felt better" in their spirits when we were together…even though they knew they were going to cross over, what a beautiful thing to be with that courageous soul at that moment. As the body was dying, the spirit soared and the room filled with expansiveness. It was almost as if they were all over the room. One human body could not contain this due to our earthly existence and having to meet requirements and deadlines. Well, at the end, it IS a dead line and the buck stops there! What a privilege it has been to experience that knowledge! To the same effect, when a baby comes into the world, we see them as fragile. We see a helpless little body... and when we see the baby open his/her eyes, our hearts jump for joy! We are still, however, not aware that the baby is more alive than we can imagine. This child has a knowing larger than we can conceive and remembers clearer, senses stronger, and sees differently than we do. We have been conditioned. Babies have not. So even our understanding of what our eyes have showed us about these little innocent beings is an illusion.

~ CONCEPTIONS IN AWAKENING ~

When standing in stillness, we wouldn't necessarily stop and consider the concept at hand called," standing in the moment of Truth." However, it's the desert that offers as much nutrient as the ocean... and stillness might be looked at like the dessert. When we learn to turn within, we open and allow ourselves to become the change. Ironically, no thought has to be involved... just be. This is where answers lie. This actually goes beyond ANY thought that you could possibly think would help your mind to ease, or find solutions to a situation, etc.

You will find that meditation is meant for this purpose. Dreaming is meditation on a higher level. When we wake up in the morning, we may feel different, even if we don't remember our dreams. The saying," She woke up on the wrong side of the bed" indicates an attitude observed that this person can hopefully realize, then will either decide to shift her reality or not. Our old patterns are being challenged now more than ever before. As we break through these old paradigms of thought processes and belief systems, we can trust (oh no…it's the "T" word!) that we are opening ourselves to allow the shift to take place within us. We think we have learned so much. Learning doesn't come in 1 form; it comes from hundreds… moment by moment. And in these moments, the speed of light to illumination occurs! We just need to be silent and listen.

~ THE LIGHT WE ARE ~

When we flip on a light switch, we get results. When we get an "A-HA" moment, we *feel* results. Our intent of our desire around that keeps the light switched on.

All thought form is connected to an electrical current that runs deep within… it's the nervous system at work. This is what its true purpose in our physical body really is. The light we live is the power we are, and by choosing the depth of illumination, knowing we have barely touched the surface, we can enhance our lives beyond measure.

Just think how much is out there we haven't experienced?? For those of us who have been through the toughest of times, we feel we can say," Man, I can tell you a thing or two"… however, what *didn't* you see in the reasons why you had to go through that tough time in the first place? There's always room for new understandings and growth. This is where we shine brighter. It's when we see more lessons for ourselves… minus the attitude. That is how we learn the lesson.

My daughter sent me a birthday card that had a Buddha on the front of it. Inside, it said "Have a great birthday and a new "Buddha-tude!"

That wonderful saying, "Once you've opened your eyes, you can't look back." If you should come past this situation again, you will recognize it and move beyond it. This process also provides you with a release of a pattern that has been there for a very long time. We all have known people, or even become someone who continually repeated the same patterns…such as, the same type of partner, or the same lesson in job hunting. Maybe not being able to stand up for ourselves when we know down deep inside we do NOT like that job, but we take it because it pays well. In the true sense of the word, why would we spend a major portion of our life doing something we know is harmful to our desires? Temporary measures are lessons as well. Yet, finding ourselves doing something we do not really enjoy creates a lack of energy that makes us age, begins depression, or worse, causes a cancer because we stayed with something we truly hated down deep.

Illumination is clearly about waking up and changing the perspective from how we've seen things to being open enough to find how much more we haven't seen.

In the movie," The Matrix", could Neil have known he was the "chosen one'? Chances are, no, not until he proved himself and moved out of fear. What does the term "chosen" mean, anyway?? Doesn't it always come down to our decisions of how far we are going to lead ourselves without the blockages of insecurity?? I wonder if Jesus or Buddha would have considered themselves chosen.

Waking up is not just with thought. (even though we have a thousand thoughts a day!) It's about stepping out of a blockage of time and limitation that we created, and reconsidering a new direction. This can be with the comments you make, the choices you're making minute by minute on a daily basis, and even your business profession.

We are in a brand new period of time. The collapses and shifts all over the world are speaking directly to us as a mirror. It is truly time to "let go" and go with the flow of New Creations! To stay healthy we must remain in balance. In the movie "Avatar", we saw that Nature's first priority was balance. In the physical body, we call it *homeostasis*.

The saying, "All things in moderation" also means we relate it to our emotional responses, our mental concepts, and our very ideas...We can achieve this balance inside ourselves, no matter who we are. We just need the virtue of listening.

Listening requires patience. It requires silence. It IS the going within that brings about a sense of serenity and calm. Simple actions are loud... like listening to an ocean... a person speaking without us giving the automated response of reaction! This is the ticket to how we create balance inside on a deep level. When we can listen, and not be or feel threatened to "what" we are hearing, that's moving forward. Standing up for oneself is truly happening with or without another person having to know it. Many times, I've seen what others are like due to insecurity. (It's my job) It's then that I get quieter. It's like a patience sign in my mind goes off and the sign flashes in neon lights! This person might be strong, when they are really scared. (this affects the circulatory system...."blood boiling") They may be shy, when down deep they have a lot to say. (throat chakra effects and immune reactions) They may be feeding me information that I can read is just not true for them, yet this is where their comfort level is still at. Listening, patience, and factual perceptions have worked for years when Spirit has something to say!

———

~ THE AGE OF INNOCENCE ~

A child of one of my clients is 5 years old. She was watching TV one night when her daddy came into the room to put her to bed. When he told her it was bedtime, her quick response was, "Daddy, there is no time." He said, "Then what are we doing here?" Her response was... "You know this father-daughter thing? Can we just be friends?" Children are like Shaman in small bodies, and in so many cases I've seen, waiting their turn to be heard!

At the ages of 5 and 6 years old, we are developing our sense of awareness to the big picture we are living in. It's not that we lose our sense of soul; it's just that we are then defining our system of how we are going to survive in the world we came into. However, many children today only have the moment. They do not necessary think about going shopping for groceries, where their next meal will come from, or even when will tomorrow be here? Why would they? They have a sense of time that in the moment, they are making their reality happen. This is why the memories of a tot that age will be more significant in later years. They were there. If the pain in the adult life is strong, so many times it's because as children, we felt who was there when the fever hit.
Who helped us ride our bikes, etc. If your memories were good, and you had a loving family, you will remember your Christmas mornings, the smell of dinner that your mom cooked when she made your favorite meal, etc. Memories determine your future, whether positive or not, we usually allow them on a subconscious level because that's all we know.

Many people are talking about living in the moment today. Actually, it's Quantum Physics that taught us that there is NO time, and there is only that which we create. Therefore, if this is true, then the good news is that we can change the memories that we created just by not attaching to them as reality…especially if we hold on to them and determine the rest of our lives by them. This is why there is hypnosis. To really dive in to memories can heal us, and it can also hurt us. Those clients of mine who are aware of very hard or sad memories can determine their future through allowing the release of the importance of that memory to exist. For example, one time I had someone who had lost her mother at the age of 3. It was her and her sister who lived with their dad. She always wondered what it would be like to have had her mother there. So we played a little trick on the mind, and as I ran energy through her body, I suggested she see her mom there during her years of important events in her life. Even though you cannot bring mom back physically, her mind saw her mother there, and eased her into fulfilling a moment that changed the way she felt all of these years. Loss and sadness in regards to this turned into saying, "It's like I feel her presence again", and that changed the way she interpreted life as a mother herself. It was in her perception. We can all see what we want to, and the feeling is what heals us. In her case, it was the satisfaction of feeling the release of that constant pain and wonderment turn into comfort, nurturing, and love.

Can we change the past? Yes, inside of our hearts, we can. Will that change the future? Certainly it can. Time and space are only significant to *us*; therefore, we can change it in seconds just by mere allowance of a new perception. This, on many levels, is why age itself is not necessarily the reason we die. When we are at an older age, and we have been healthy from all aspects in life, our organs can give out of course. However for the most part, we reach a stage in life where we can now actually advance and *move on* by what we call…death. Even in death, our perceptions can lift us into higher realms of frequency on the other side. Again, time over there doesn't exist, and the more we are able to let go of this linear thinking, the freer we become.

When swimming with dolphins on the Big Island in Hawaii, I caught the eye of a mother with her baby mimicking her every move right alongside of her. Her eye said "we're connected" to me in a second… so I followed them. At what I thought was only 5 minutes of swim time next to them, turned out to be 45 minutes. Finally realizing I had swam so fast, that when I dropped back to our earthly reality, no one was out in the ocean where I ended up! Fascinating experience when you realize that you were basically taken out of a consciousness where there is no space or time. It was as if I was flying and lost all sense of direction and time, and didn't even care whatsoever.

There is not a thing that is set in stone, no matter what your belief systems are, or for that matter, how you perceive anything. This is why being open and living every day as though it is totally new, is a "free-way" into being! People have asked me if a baby is waiting in the wings before a pregnancy occurs. I don't like to burst anyone's bubble, but the answer is no with all of the reads I've done. It is not until a soul decides to enter that the decision becomes reality. We, as humans, do not see beyond our physical realities at times, so when we try to understand the process of how life works, somehow it feels better to categorize it, or say it is a certain way. Illumination includes spontaneous moments and allowance for something new and different to occur in any given situation. There is the joy and the adventure!

I will tell you about one incident that happened when I was working one day about 12 years ago. A woman came to see me that was 5 months pregnant. Her mom was a regular client of mine, and fortunately sent her daughter in for a session. This daughter had not been pregnant before. So when she came in to the healing room, little did we BOTH know what was going to happen next!

I asked her if she had ever had an energy session before of any kind. She said no, but decided it sounded pretty neat with what her mother was experiencing in her sessions with me. This gal drove quite a ways for this. So as I started working on her stomach, I immediately read that there was no life in this baby. I asked the woman how long had it been since her last checkup. Her answer was 2 weeks ago. So at this point, I looked up to the heavens and asked "Why did you send her to me?" I then felt the need to put my hands on her belly, one hand on the baby's feet and the other on the head. Of course, this was a 5 month pregnancy, so my hands practically moved themselves into the position necessary for me to run the energy necessary. Even I wasn't sure what would happen here. The energy from my hands began to not only heat up, but permeate dramatically through this lovely lady who was seriously conking out fast! This was good, because for whatever was to happen, the energy was acting like an anesthesia to a degree. As I sat with my hands in this position, I felt a major surge go through *my* body! It felt like I was knocked off balance and my equilibrium took a few minutes to get back. Within about 2 minutes, I felt a kick from this little baby right under my right hand. I felt a huge sense of relief as the mother then said with a groggy sounding comment, "Oh, there it is." Shocked and elated at the same time, I continued as though nothing big had just happened. I certainly wasn't going to blurt out, "Hey! Now your baby has a life!" This was a miracle, if you will. A moment in time that only I knew…well, me and that soul!

I finished the session, said good bye to my client, and then went to the restroom to find myself strongly feeling a sense of sadness that had me crying pretty hard. After 5 minutes, I dried my eyes and started on the next person.

A week later, I had gone to have my own session with my wonderful Cherokee mentor. I asked her to tell me what happened, as Karen could read energy no matter what it was. She told me that one of my guides had surged out of me and into the baby's body so it could live here now. No wonder I cried so hard. The loss of losing a guide that quickly left me feeling a bit weak and empty. To this day, I was told by Spirit that I would not be able to see this child in this life. I had the opportunity 7 years later when my original client found me in my new location. She had informed me that the little boy was doing well, and the energy I read during the session of this

baby all happened. His labor was difficult, and yes, he was a piano player. When I snuck in the question as to whether or not I could see him, she said her daughter lived nearby and she would tell her I was at this new location, leaving me hopeful. Yet, if he would have seen me, it would be obvious the boy would feel very drawn to wanting to come home with me, and maybe that could have disrupted their lives, etc. Spirit was working in our favor when I realized I would not see him this lifetime. As sad as it made me at the time, the cycle of life had its own fabulous plan, and I was blessed to be a part of it.

7.

Quantum and Indigenous
~ Facts and Knowledge ~

"Humankind has not woven the web of life. We are but one thread within it. Whatever we do to the web, we do to ourselves. All things are bound together. All things connect." Chief Seattle 1854~

I am not a scholar in Quantum Physics with a degree in science or quantum mechanics. However, all that I have learned has been from "hands-on" experience and BEING that which these scholars talk about…. if you know what I mean! When understanding that we carry indigenous grids and memory in our very own blood, our bodies, and our remembrance of the past, we must truly know that there is nothing stopping the flow of this connected knowledge to *anyone*. We are simply re-remembering information that existed somewhere in our blood many lifetimes ago. Energy begets energy. Therefore, we are inherent with memory as we come back to this world to begin again the lessons of growth in order to achieve a higher frequency of living… a better life with wisdom. Transference, osmosis, conscious creation and evolutionary patterns from the past are all a part of us and our growth.

When I was in my early teens, I watched a program on TV that related to the queen of Mongolia. She was buried in a valley in the hills of Mongolia with 12 horse heads surrounding her grave. I do not remember who was digging up the grave; however, it didn't seem to matter. The point being that my soul almost jumped out of my own body because it was so auspicious to me. My skin developed goose bumps and my recognition of memory kicked in. I began to physically have a reaction in that I recognized that queen to be me. I literally became aware of the knowledge of who I was at that time. Since I am a reader of energy and have been my whole life, this sent me into a chill and shock to my current system. So instead of becoming afraid of it, I became one with it and read the memory of her bones as they dug the grave up and opened the coffin. I saw the jewelry that was familiar to me. I also was able to determine why they buried me there. It was sacred land and I was well liked and respected as their queen.

Many years later, when I met my mentor, Cherokee seer, Karen Land, I did not speak of this. Instead, I had asked her about my past lives at one time. Our conversation was so real and so very resonant to my being. She confirmed that I was a Mongolian queen that had been buried with 12 horse heads around my grave.

One life always leads to another. I like to consider this life like a calendar. We turn the pages, but it's the same year. Each day can also be considered a life time now with how fast things seem to be moving! The Shaman know that there is no time and that one life leads to another to continue the process of undeniable desire to get to return to Spirit one day whole and complete.

Quantum reality is based in true awareness of fact when science tells us that it's the space in between the cells that carries the essence of life and actually dictates life into form…the cell. It becomes a virtual fact that these spaces hold the memory of all things happening in the body, and the cells become the conduits in order to perform what that information is. This is why we have the right and the means to change anything in ourselves any time we choose.

(just like a Genie in a bottle…) Not everyone needs to know their past lives; however, if there is a block in the current growth, chances are it might be a little harder than originally thought to advance. This is why we must be honest with ourselves through our emotions. This is the best way to advance. Again, where two or more are gathered and confrontation through growth occurs, we can step into a new awareness and see life as a huge chapter being written by you.

It isn't so much the necessity to rediscover where you have walked, as much as it is to go face to face with a lesson waiting to teach you the essence of the bliss you desire today, giving you permission to become enlightened through humility and expansiveness. This is the key to happiness.

A four year old child came in with a fever. He was incredibly smart, and very cute! We spoke of this fever, and I told him I would be speaking to him like an adult. I explained his fever was about the anger he was carrying due to his brother not loving him the way he expected he should. He looked at me with those big beautiful brown eyes and said "You are right on." I had him explain to me what he thought his brother should be doing different. Once he got the feelings out of his system, we talked about how his brother needed a little space but he didn't love him any less. As I worked on his little body to get the cough to alleviate, (congestion is due to confusion of how to feel) he looked at me and said that he could only imagine how fun things would be very soon. I applauded this little sweetie and reminded him as long as he didn't forget to see the reason *why* he got sick in the first place, and then he would get well and have fun.

I gave a talk on "Health Care for Today" recently when a lady from the audience came up to me and called me a "Quantum Shaman." I giggled and then decided that the title was appropriate, considering the understanding of cosmic correlation between our Spirit and our physical body.

~ THE PROPHET IN YOU ~

Prophets of the past have been able to read the future. This is truly special and highly unique to those times when Nostradamus was alive. You can't have prophesy or any read without accepting the larger picture that there is so much more that we are now tapping in to. These prophets knew this. The truth is that *anyone can do this.* People believe you have to be born gifted in order to produce wowed effects. This simply is not true. Many people are coming into more of their own wisdom and hearing themselves saying things to other people that they didn't even know they knew! All it takes is pure desire and less negative talk about themselves and others. This alone changes the old patterns that have not been recognized by us, and keeps us more open to possibilities with ourselves. It is as if we are emptying the bucket and cleaning it out in order to retain more. More and more people are also beginning to see that they recognize places that look familiar on some level, even though they have not been there in this life. Many of our children born today are mentioning this to their parents without any hesitation.

The indigenous healers and Shaman have always known that there is no stopping the flow of God or energy that they accept as Oneness.

The only ones who stop any form of creation is us.

We have the free will to see things however we want to, limited or not. The choice will always be ours to allow or disallow. The more knowledge we accept as possibilities and truths, the more we let go and make it happen. The Shamans embody truth in themselves in order to produce truth in others. They don't have to say a word. They just are. Their presence alone fills a room with a feeling of awe or even hope. If you've ever attended a pow wow, then you know the purpose is for celebration and connection. What better form than dance to describe and express every cell appreciating life? This is respect at the highest level. Trance states have certainly been reached. I have seen some dancers that continually dance in high temperatures with all the regalia for hours and hours at a time. They are immersed in a type of trance state that allows them to keep going. Their intent is strictly love beyond their own ego. This transcendence overrides the fact that their bodies are so tired or so hot. At that point, they do not give that any relevance and they just keep going. Their gift to their Creator is that of oneness in and throughout their blood.

When you walk into a place where there are elders, you naturally feel the respect all throughout the area. We have had the 13 Grandmothers appearing for many to witness as they travel around the globe. What is their message? Peace and truth to all. They are providing a wake up call to humanity through song and healing and prayer being their intent. The ancients long ago are being acknowledged today for their sharp wisdom over thousands of years. If we didn't find this of any interest, then why would there be all of this commotion about the "end of times as we've known them" on December 21st, 2012?

In the world known as Indigenous, we automatically think of traditional tribes performing rituals to suit their beliefs and their way of connection. It is true, however, that the Shaman of these tribes become much, much more than just *only* a part of his or her tribal connection. They become a light to the world through the oneness of their spirit *to* the Earth and with the Divine. It is where Humanity is going. All of us are beginning to take note on this deep level of expansion within ourselves, and it is definitely creating a sense of Unity, called Consciousness. Or as I like to phrase it, we are now in the time of "Shamanizing Humanity."

~ My Personal Story as a Shaman ~

I have been attracted to, lived, seen, worked with, and loved Indigenous Medicine Shaman most of my life. I have always wanted to be an elder, since I can remember. I sat with mother on the porch one day at the age of 7 and said to her, "You must be real happy at your age." She looked at me very curious like, and then she replied, "What do you mean?" I told her I wanted to be her age and then get the benefits of discounts on groceries, etc. She laughed and then she said, "You are one weird child!" I just smiled.

At the age of 5, I remember watching a movie on TV about Jesus on the cross. I couldn't take my eyes off of it. I sat practically right ON the TV when my mom asked me to scoot back. I told her," I know him." Of course, she responded with a statement of how absurd that was. Then my response back to her was, "Do you know how he stayed alive for three hours up there?" She said, "No, smarty pants, how *did* Jesus stay alive for three hours up there?" I responded, "He knew how to move his feet." I immediately knew that he could move his feet to keep the circulation moving, even with a nail in them that kept him alive for the time he had.

After those A-HA moments, I began to realize that I came back to Earth to do the work I chose. When in Sunday school one day, I looked down at my hands and couldn't believe how wrinkled they were at the age of 10. I noticed my teachers' hands and other ladies had beautiful hands... even my sisters. Why were mine so wrinkled? I received information at that moment that they were very old hands. They had lots more work to do. So I accepted them and, being in Sunday school, agreed they were OK, and yes, they'd do just fine!

At 19 years old, I heard of an organization called the Jesuit Volunteer Corp from my dad who did business cards for a priest in San Francisco. I was so happy to be accepted, even without the mandatory degree they requested with the application. I was chosen to be an Activity Director for 4 senior citizen centers in Juneau, Alaska. My experience with the Klinket Indian shut-ins was extremely gratifying. To sit down with these beautiful people and listen to their stories at the age of 20, was beyond what I ever could have read in a book. They shared their Native way of the heart, and they were so real, I didn't want to leave them. I'd come back with food driving the "senior limousine" the next day and do it all over again! This went on for a year. The day I got married, I had received a package at my door. When I looked to see who it was from, it was one of my favorite and wise Klinket elders who, at that time, taught me about what it was like to be blind. She died 2 months before her daughter had found the package in a room that had been addressed to me. It was incredibly touching to know that I had made such a difference in her life. I felt like she didn't die at all! She bought me the towels I had commented on the last time I had seen her. She was gone, but not really.

Years later, I was introduced to my mentor, a Cherokee Seer and amazing healer, Karen Land. She had been recommended to me to see from a friend who had heard of her awesome ability to run energy in the body. Being curious, I made the appointment, and my life has never been the same. I was fortunate to have learned from her in every way for 12 years. Her wisdom touched hundreds of people, and the truth through her hands is where I learned much of the knowledge I've gained. I asked her once what the Bible meant when the Book of Revelations spoke of the "beast." Who or what was this beast? Her answer, simply stated, was, "Well honey, the beast is the ego." That was enough for me. She was quick, sharp, and took me on as her student 24-7. I was on the hot seat more than once, but it was worth every second. The Cherokee keep their word, and she did!

When she passed in 2005, I had developed the symptoms of her last physical condition in *my* body, and knew I needed a Shaman to be high enough in vibration to help me rid this. I had a client at that time that was so grateful for the work he'd received, that he and his wife sent me a first class ticket to Hawaii. I had wanted to go to Hawaii for so long, and never found the time or made the time to go. It happened when I most needed it through this wonderful client... and when I went to Hawaii to stay with them, I asked the client if he knew of any Kupuna in the area (a wise Hawaiian elder with the gift of healing hands). Fortunately, he did, and meeting this Kupuna was the beginning of my knowledge with the Sacred Hawaiian healing and tradition. I studied under him for almost a year as an ala kai student to this sacred healing. Lomi lomi wasn't just a form of massage; it was the way in which a true Hawaiian elder was able to interpret or see the body and work on many areas of dysfunction. I realized this must have been my life before because I did this automatically in my work from the start!

I found so many Massage Therapists on the mainland could not explain this meaning, no matter who I'd ask. They stumbled at their own responses. It wasn't until I found the beauty myself in what this meant that the answer was given. In Hawaiian healing, we have much more than Lomi Lomi. There is the knowledge of the plants and herbs such as the ti leaf. Each plant offers something... and it's the ancients that knew the benefits of them. It is the study of "Lapa au."(herbs). These deep Shaman (Kahuna to some, even though that word does not have the same meaning as it did years ago) healers understood that greeting each other was most respectfully done with the "Ha" breath. This is a greeting given from

Hawaiian to Hawaiian in the form of breath to each other. Two Hawaiians will put their foreheads together and make the exhale into a whisper of "Ha." They won't usually kiss at this type of greeting. It becomes the meaning of love, caring, respect, joy, and long life simply in one breath. When witnessed, it's awe-some.

It isn't just the people who are ancients. The Earth has many loved ones under her wing that are just as profound. Volcanoes for example…

If you ever have heard of the Goddess Pele, the legend is tremendous. She is known as the Kilauea Volcano in Hilo, on the Big Island of Hawaii. Thousands of people flock to the island to see her luscious lava pour into the ocean, as well as enjoy the beauty and peace in a land of enchantment. It is said that if you take a lava rock from her without asking, your life will have many significant reactions that are not positive experiences! This is true.

When I was studying with my Kupuna, he used to tell me that Pele's love was like a precious grandmother (which is where she developed the name "Tutu Pele"). I saw that he had a great affiliation to her personality, and this fascinated me. There is a center at the Volcano National Park where people return stones because their lives had gone awry. But this just made me more excited about meeting Pele. The Kupuna had mentioned that when you come home to Hawaii, Pele gets very happy to have her grandchild back. It does not matter if it's this life, or one where she knew you before. The feeling I had when I first laid eyes on her was unlike any feeling I ever experienced. One day, the Kupuna was having trouble physically. I knew I could work with him to do a great healing. However, he was plagued with Diabetes, and had a recent operation where he lost his leg. So I went to the Volcano National Park and spoke to Pele. Much to my surprise, she and I developed an instant love for each other, and she began to blow wind my way. It got undeniably strong. My inner voice was calm and I began to listen. I started hearing words in the wind. (So THIS is what the Native Americans mean when we "listen to the wind!") She told me to go back and tell the Kupuna that he must act within the laws of Aloha. "True to Self" is the term we use, called "Pono." She told me a few things I didn't even read as an energy runner. I was surprised, yet relieved that I could go back and tell him. He heard it.

Well, this became rather addicting to know that I could tune in and hear her when she wanted to talk to me. When Pele is listening to your request and accepts your gifts of flowers or fruit, she will show as a white bird going solo in the crater. She flies so magnificently that you cannot help but know the grace of her beauty.

So I went back once a week for one year, expressing my love through chanting, singing (mele), and listening to her marvelous wisdom. I left to come back to the mainland after my training was complete on October 14th, 2006. The fumes of the vog (volcano fog) were beginning to get strong the morning before I went to say goodbye. On October 13th, early in the morning, I looked out over the crater and realized something was not right. The bird did not show. So I waited about 15 minutes and told Pele that I refused to leave until I saw the bird and knew she was alright. Two minutes passed, and the bird flew sideways in the crater. She had shown herself, but then something strange happened! The bird disappeared right before my eyes. It was there, then it was gone. I waited a few minutes, and she re-appeared again just to do the same. I realized I was stubborn, but this was Pele's way of telling me it was time to go. I had to make sure she was all right. Yet, because Pele is all about respect, I listened and walked away with a sad heart.

It was the hardest thing I ever did, but I knew I would be back when it was time. Pele would call me in my heart. I knew I would feel it. Midnight came and I was on a plane back to the West Coast. I was traveling with a dear friend whom I looked at before we entered the plane and I said, "If 9/11 had happened here, would you still call this paradise??" We boarded right after that.

I arrived to my destination six hours later to hear the televisions in the airport blurting out loud that there was a 6.6 earthquake on the Big Island of Hawaii at 7 a.m. on October 14th.

~ ALOHA MAGIC ~

I went back to see Pele on October 14th, 2009…not realizing it had been three years to the day that experience had happened. I went back because I had a client give me a 10 day stay to write this book on Maui. Yet, I knew I was being "called" to go alone. I made it my retreat and spent the last four days in Hilo and Kona. I finally got to see Pele the last day I was on the Island. I knew something was up because the call was strong.

When I arrived at the Volcano National Park, I was right. When I got out of the car in the parking lot holding the orchids I had to give Pele, I fell straight down to my knees with the hardest grief I had ever experienced! I cried so spontaneously. It was like projectile vomiting. When I picked myself back up and walked over to the crater, I noticed my heart pouring love (ALOHA) and felt as though I had left her. My heart was saddened, however, because I knew this wasn't my grief. It was clearly hers.

I sat next to the crater and told Pele I was there to help in any way I could. She then showed me the beautiful white bird! The shine radiating from the wings was enough to soften that sad feeling. This was a reunion.

Then the wind blew. I consider this "the HA breath." So I blew back to her. She had me listen to the message that she needed (and wanted) me to share. This message abides today, and so I share it with you. She asked me to put her in the book.

Here is her message….

"Seven hundred and fifty thousand people have come to see me since you left me three year ago today. In that 750,000, not one has seen me. Their fear is great. They are afraid that the vog is hurting them. They are afraid of the volcano blowing up then killing them. They look the other way when a lesson can be learned and comes up for them.

I pour myself into that Ocean for the people so they can create this new land with the Aloha Spirit originally intended and bring back a land that is fresh, new, and expansive. If the people knew that this is why the lava flows now, maybe they will add their true hearts of simplicity, gratitude, and love. But they are too busy speaking of Atlantis and Lemuria. Those places became corrupt. Why do you think I buried them?"

This information was overwhelming for me at that moment. So that explained why I was called to listen and cry with her at that time.

Permission and respect are of utmost importance in Hawaii, and everywhere else on Earth. When taking a lava rock, as long as you ask permission, and you do it with love, then it becomes a gift of the land to you. The honored respect of which giving and receiving occurs is the balance of the land and the people being one. Pele pours graciousness and peace in her lava flow. We need to pay attention. With fear, we not only find ourselves blocking deeper connections, but we also find ourselves resisting the highest form of love one could possibly have.

~ THE CONNECTION ~

The quantum aspect of healing is allowing a change in our belief systems with respect to knowledge that we haven't learned yet. Knowing that there is always more makes us feel as though we are like new babies with potentials and dynamic abilities we haven't even touched yet. How exciting to realize that one shifted perception can change the world. I know this is a lot to comprehend; however, if you consider that quantum thought has no time then that leaves the door wide open for possibilities. This, then, is how we continue to move forward in a world by contributing to it....not being run by it. As Jesus so eloquently phrased it, "I am in the world, not of it." Being in higher frequencies, we can now say we are almost ready as a collective unit in this school of humanity, to be in it *and* of it as our consciousness rises as a whole. Whether we understand it or not, we are becoming a collective in the realm of quantum thought and instant manifestation. I feel so inspired when I remember the stories of Christ. I do feel that this is what Jesus's purpose was from the beginning. Who knows? Maybe this IS the second coming? The Christ consciousness in action!

My recently deceased business partner, John Jay Harper, loved going on radio to share his insights into the future, and people loved his sweet voice of wisdom. He wrote the following paragraph for a new book he had been writing:

"When we look through the lens of microscopes and telescopes we see there are no boundaries to creation; we are a soup, thus, in the final analysis we are not and cannot be separate from each other, nature, or God. There is only one source of intelligence underlying reality that we call the vacuum of space, or the zero-point field. The implication is that we are immortal beings of light that come and go through a membrane made of consciousness itself lifetime after lifetime."

John passed away on December 15th, 2010. Our hearts were connected as close friends who "got it" when we were talking at length for six hours at a time without getting up once for any reason. Our very connection alone was magnificent, and as energy proves to not know distance, we had a shared death experience, as author Raymond Moody of the book, Life after Life explains. "A shared death experience is stronger than a near death experience for the one left behind." I can certainly attest to that. Spiritual experiences are happening more and more as time gets stronger in the new paradigm of living. As 2012 continues to unfold, we are being given a gift. It means that this is the time of change, of fortune, of unraveling the past, We are seeing our issues brought up in order to release them. On a personal note, I feel this is the best year ever. It is the true beginning of our future of interpersonal relationships with like-minded people to create a unity of conscious teamwork. Or better yet, a community of people who are mastering their love for each other by living directly from their hearts. (The heart of the matter is truly the matter of the heart) This is the wave of the future by terms of the Indigenous and by terms of Science. With organizations such as Heartmath, director Howard Martin teaches us the direct magnification of our human heart and the connection to the Earth, the Solar Flares, and each other. We have no reason to discount this epic opportunity to unite.

What is the difference then in Indigenous concepts and understandings vs. scientific facts and comprehension? It's one and the same. There is no difference. However, the energy force that drives a Shaman to that knowledge is gratitude and recognition of conscious oneness. That leads to wisdom and gracious humility. That leads to happiness, and then our cells know that through our shifting, we are one with all things. Energy runs our world. We can transmute anything. This is known as snake medicine according to some

Native American traditions. We are learning that we are shedding our old skin (patterns, thoughts, limited belief systems, etc.) on a personal and global level. Now, if we can combine that knowledge with the knowing of *where two or more are gathered*, we will then see that the energy of one is one, two is two hundred, three is three thousand, and so on. Truthfully, this is how we can change the world together and create back the bountiful and once luscious planet, to call Heaven on Earth. In the eyes of a Shaman, we feel *connected* to all things. We respect the land, our tribe and mostly, our self. Without that we might as well not be Shaman. When we speak of raising Consciousness we are really saying that our internal world must be whole and complete, as we know we cannot sufficiently live without nature. You might say we become a Universe within ourselves and create a harmonic frequency when we do this together. This alone initializes peace and oneness and that brings about more peace and oneness.

Quantum facts are not judgments. They are precisely correct and can change any amount of energy in seconds. Energy healing can be better understood from this way of viewing. This is why it is so important to understand that our perceptions are mutable and can change an entire planet from being in chaos and separation to being all related and united.

8.

~ The Galactic Human ~

"Doctors don't know everything! They understand matter, not spirit. You and I live in spirit."
~William Saroyan , *The Human Comedy*

We are at a time of dramatic change, not only in ourselves, but in the world and even the Universe.

Most of us have already discovered that these changes are affecting the ways we live, think, and make decisions, which have been based on concepts we figured were working for us before. With major economic changes alone, we are questioning what's next for the Global community as well as for our own families. The "Clarion Call" for awakening to awareness in 2012 is advancing at such a rate that seems unprecedented. Yet the feeling of change is light, and the drifting away of our old ways of living and thinking is allowing us to be free of our past, both individually and through our behaviors globally. We are doing this in the form of *Consciousness.*

In the book called <u>The Gaia Project</u>, by Hwee-Yong Jang, translated by Mira Tyson, it states that "Consciousness can be defined as a faculty of a being who perceives the world and creates something out of that perception. From this viewpoint, the nature of being, including that of the human beings, can be described as consciousness." I love that definition of Consciousness, mainly because it indicates that perception is the guiding force of where we lead ourselves and gives new meaning to the phrase "*As within, so without.*" The conscious brain sits in our prefrontal cortex. It is responsible for our creativity and has no perception of time. It doesn't hang on to our personal identity and is capable of shifting reality into non-reality. Actually, it is what really gives us empowerment, or not.

The subconscious mind is in the rest of the brain and lives in the present moment. It doesn't understand creation the way the conscious mind does because it identifies itself as the big picture. We minimize this and turn it into *creation* through the conscious mind. That is what makes us co-creators in the vastness of life itself. It is what gives us our personal choices in order to live in a way we can understand. The sub-conscious doesn't see the same way the conscious does, so this is where we can become more aware of our personal contribution to life.

My business partner in 2010 was an Author, a Scientist, and a Visionary. He was one of the most passionate men I have ever met, a true genius when it came to understanding Life, Love, God, the Polar Shift, and the Human Race. We could sit together and converse on deep subjects for six hours at a time without ever having to leave our seats for any reason. John Jay Harper wrote the book entitled <u>Transformers; Shaman of the 21st Century</u>. I found out later that he had been on the Internet radio program <u>Coast to Coast</u> several times as well as several other radio shows. We met quite spontaneously one day when we were on Facebook. He sought help for a condition in his neck that he thought was from a car accident forty years prior. His ears rang relentlessly, and the pain in his neck was indescribable. He had tried all of the alternative methods for help and had resorted to medical drug therapy. This didn't work either. Nothing he found was able to relieve the ringing or the pain.

He invited me to his home in Spokane, Washington, where I met his wife, daughter, and grandchildren. The day I met John at the airport, we felt as though we have always known each other, therefore, I enjoyed my three- day stays in

July and again in August of 2010. I had explained my work to John before I met him. I told him I could energetically read him, his past, and his thoughts, for that matter. Mostly, I could read his pain. He cried very hard the first time I worked on him. I saw the memory of his mother walking by his crib…like seeing through John's eyes when he was 2 years old. I saw her legs, but never did I see or feel John getting picked up. Immediately I knew he was going through abandonment. He not only discussed this with me, but was shocked how right on I was with seeing the vision. {He then shared with many people that he found there to be much healing when truth is revealed through the muscle. Yet we are still, and always will be, ultimately responsible for our own healing.}

This, then, was one reason I feel that his pain came back in the form of ringing in the ears and nerve dysfunction. John began to feel less pain toward the last month he was here on this planet. However, he wasn't afraid of passing at all. John's fascination with NDE's (near death experiences) continued to expand as he himself was getting ready for the next adventure.

His writings on the topic of health included many quotes from many authors, including Joseph Campbell, author of <u>The Power of Myth</u> and <u>An Open Life</u>. He enjoyed quoting the Bible and also musical artists. He quoted Huey Lewis and the News singing, "We need a new drug, one that won't make us sick." He and I spoke of Humanity needing to wake up to what real health was all about, something we were both willing to share together. We were the Scientist and the Shaman coming together to teach how to upgrade our DNA software file codes and brain hardware circuits for life in the 21st Century. Now that John is gone, I am moved to abide by his request and write the book that has been inside me throughout my entire life. We both made an agreement that everything we did together would be 50/50. This partnership ranged from talks, books, and CD's to radio programs, which we would begin in February, 2011. Now I include his awesome information in this book to keep my end of the bargain!

Many people on Facebook and friends and family were looking forward to our work. Yes, I must say, we had a knack for sharing insights! When John's wife Connie generously allowed me to go through John's information and take what I felt pertinent to share after he passed, I collaborated with what his best writings and teachings entailed. He would have wanted all of us to know his scientific and visionary understandings for 2012 and beyond. Some of what I am about to share is also about the Earth and the lead-in to the current Polar Shift we are now experiencing. John passed in late 2010, so keep in mind that he wasn't here in 2011. I will point out that he wanted everyone to understand the importance of living at heart center. We taught this, similar to what we hear now with HeartMath, Gregg Braden, and many other wonderful teachers in our world today. Our future existence is and will be more based directly from our hearts. We will think from our heart center as we feel answers merge with the thoughts as an after effect. The mind makes a terrible employer but does very well as an employee!

~ A HOLOGRAPHIC PROJECTION ~

Because John was a scientist in all of his great understandings of facts and knowledge, I loved asking him questions. One sunny afternoon on his deck, we were enjoying a conversation about holograms. I asked him if his idea of a hologram was different than the dictionary's, mainly because the dictionary was brief. (I chuckle here because John was anything but brief!) He said that hologram meant, "Whole message." The whole is in the part and the part is in the whole. So when it came to discussing Universal facts, he said the Universe is actually a holographic projection. From a personal standpoint, the hologram is the way we see through our mind's eye (the 3rd eye). Holography, then, is the way the brain processes electromagnetic information through the nervous system, which creates images in the brain. We convert a signal of information into an image, and this is how we perceive life.

We live in a multi-dimensional reality. Everything that can exist does exist. We seem to be tuned to a **human** perception of reality. This can make things seem strange if we don't understand, for example, why we have dreams that don't make sense. It's what is called the *bleed through* of other dimensions seeping into our personal consciousness. From other realities, we are able to tap into dreamtime. The Shaman knows that dreamtime is sacred and respected as a way of communication from Spirit for our highest good. We wouldn't be tapping in to something so magnificent and vast unless we had the capacity to expand, and on some level, to understand this in our own consciousness. Therefore, our dreams are real. We know this from waking up with a sense of realism from another world. So, as John described, in order to make something real, either consciously or subconsciously, we would have to mentally allow willpower to play a part in this. (Now here's where it gets a little scientific, but I'll explain it in layman's terms in the best way to understand what is happening today.)

This introduces the concept and reality of *magnetics*. We're talking about ley lines and song lines, grid lines in the earth which are similar to meridians of the physical body. Magnetics draw out to what is like it and can vibrate at the same capacity. Now that we are kicking up more vibrations of the electromagnetic field, our minds are expanding. We are going into the zero point fields. We will begin to tap into these multi-dimensional realms much more as time continues. Even now we are talking about seeing angels, aliens, loved ones who have crossed, all in our scope of vision. As time continues, the realms will also include more lucid dreaming. We actually may feel drawn to a place when we wake back into *this* world, and this world will seem like the one that is *not* real.

Since we are tuning into too many frequencies at once, this may not feel *normal* to us anymore. The typical human being isn't used to all of this energy elevation. However, if we tune into this *bleed through*, we are going to create a perception of reality that is not going to match our neighbor, family members, etc. This would be considered *abnormal* by today's standards. It's time that we begin to practice "abnormal physics and paranormal psychology!"

~ WHO ARE WE? ~

"Our pineal gland is becoming activated. We need to unload our minds, realizing we are becoming impeccably aware that we are all leaders, teachers and students." ~John Jay Harper~

First of all, when we realize how much alike we are yet so individually unique, we have to see that life is actually comical in its simplicity. Now we can find ourselves giggling at the idea of judgment because we are feeling that there is no need for this type of primitive thinking, either within ourselves or in the world. Unfortunately, even though we see it continuing to occur around different parts of the world, our knowledge of this type of thinking supports the fact that judgment is losing its false power. Therefore, we will not pay heed to such a low vibration.

We are rising above the mundane as time continues to help us acknowledge the truth of our oneness. On one of John's last radio interviews, he was asked the question; "Who are we?" His eloquent style and passion proved to be profound once again when his answer stated, "We are a species now that is developing into a multi-dimensional consciousness. We are an experiment in consciousness, if you will, and are going into a field of cosmic consciousness. This means that we are going into our hearts. What the human being is doing now is waking up. We are holding hands together as we walk into this new level of reality.

We are transducers. This means we are transmitters and receivers of consciousness that is generated by the Earth, by our Solar System, and by the center of the Galaxy. We are really in a window of opportunity for the human being to tune into this Galactic Center. This sense of unity, or *at-one-ment*, with the cosmos shows us that time seems to be speeding up. For some, it is slowing down. For others, it has stopped, and we are coming into the moment of the eternal NOW that the mystics have taught us for centuries. As we become increasingly activated in this process, we will increase our awareness. We now are beginning to feel more as we *feel* our way into the future individually, and collectively."

He continued to discuss eco-location the way that dolphins process their information in their environment in the ocean. "They send a signal as we know, and they take that information as it comes off an object and is returned to their consciousness. They create an image of that. It becomes holographic in their communication."

As John continued to impress the radio host, he added many other wonderful insights as to where we are going in this newfound state of aligned consciousness with and of the Universe. He talked about the idea of telepathy that was initially a sense of mind-to-mind communication. With that said, intuition will then become a visual image. We are feeling our way into the future because the signal now is low, but as we link up with this in our minds (our mind's eye, the third eye) through the pineal gland, this image will become stronger and stronger. It will be a sense of actually turning ourselves inside out. The outside and the inside will become one side. We will see new skills coming our way.

~ AWAKENING THE PLANETARY MIND ~

Now that we are recognizing the changes on the planet and within ourselves, many of us are feeling a strange sense of emptiness or a sense of *disconnect* to who we used to be. As scary as this feels, it is right in line with the waking up process. In other words, we are feeling our way in through a new awareness as we let go of the old ideas of our identity. Many of my clients have been afraid that they are going crazy. Our thinking is being challenged because a strong sense of our future will not be led by *thinking* as we've known it. The thinking process will align with heart- centered living, and as we become more active in this state, we will begin to realize that our thoughts are like monkey chatter. Therefore, we will be able to quiet our minds much better consciously and move forward without associated fears getting in the way. One way to see these fears is to realize that certain conditions of the physical body are taking effect faster and faster as manifestation occurs at a quicker rate. Some people are being diagnosed with bi-polar disorder. Several types of personality disorders are also being diagnosed. Our stress levels are becoming higher the more we try to live the way we always have thought we needed to, in order to survive in this world. It can take us out of our comfort zones as we live in the challenge of change. As negative as it may seem, it isn't at all. It is the perception that unfamiliarity creates emptiness and a fear. Some people then react to this fear by negative behavior, such as guilt, shame, anger, blame, etc. If you have noticed these within you, just know that all of the behavior patterns that have not been dealt with within us are being amplified. However, NOW is the time to recognize that our choices are prevailing; old primitive concepts are definitely a thing of the past as we launch into more awareness. This brings with it opportunity beyond our conscious understanding, and what some would term as "magic," that is basically a form of alignment to the new creation we are becoming, individually and collectively.

Many people are talking about a Polar Shift happening today and for the next few years. If we read Gregg Braden's book <u>Deep Truth</u>, we will see that he has depicted cycles that have been occurring on our planet and in the Solar System for thousands of years. He states, "We appeared on Earth, looking as we do today, 200,000 years --30 world-age cycles and two ice ages ago." He tells us that our bodies bear the unmistakable signs of an intelligent design. This we know from eons of time being here on Earth, so now we need to wake the process more into this intelligence through the understanding of our real, true power.

Planets, just like us, have recurring patterns as they rotate and offer another go around. However, we are now in a conscious position of being able to align with this particular timing and change as our loving Universe gives us the encouragement with the momentum of *full speed ahead*. Instead of resisting our intelligence, maybe this time, we can understand. Oneness occurring in this cycle can change our present 3rd dimensional living into a 5th dimensional awareness of Divine interaction into freedom.

Consciousness, or Spirit, is a magnetic phenomenon. Living in the physical body alone doesn't make sense when we know now that we are the driver of the vehicle through our thoughts, mental creativity, and perceptions of our own realities. This is why so many authors of NDE's, (near death experiences) are enjoying teaching us and describing the death process as a phenomenon of feeling, such as being pulled out of the body like a magnetic iron filing. Even the Law of

Attraction is a magnetic phenomenon: Likes attract; opposites repel. So where we are now, and where we are continuing to go, is magnetic in itself. When electricity and magnetics unite, we have an electromagnetic occurrence; Our Solar flares today are enhancing this effect within us, individually and collectively, and helping the old to become new. Therefore, knowing that a Pole Shift is occurring helps us to realize that it is an electromagnetic shift that is bringing back the electrical and magnetic component of the Earth, which is opening the floodgates of consciousness.

It is crucial for our unity to be understood and lived. As a human race given all potential to be one unit, work as one unit, and achieve splendor in our hearts and souls, it is imperative now to accept this ultimate blessing and change the world. The Constitution of the United States says, "By the people, for the people." Now is our time to shine like never before and utilize the astrological abundance being offered. Humanity is becoming shamanized. In John's words, "We are becoming conscious now of being co-creators of a new heaven and a new earth. Whatever we can create, we can manifest. Whatever we can create, we *will* manifest!"

Made in the USA
San Bernardino, CA
28 February 2017